PLANT BASED C

A Guide On How To Switch To A Plant Based Diet As A Beginners, Kids, Athletes And Families With Transforming Recipe

By

Williams Cook

Copyright © 2020 Williams Cook

All rights reserved. No part of this book shall be reproduced, stored in a retrieval system, or transmitted by any means, electronic, mechanical, photocopying, recording, or otherwise, without written permission from the publisher. Although every precaution has been taken in the preparation of this book, the publisher and author assume no responsibility for errors or omissions. Nor is any liability assumed for damages resulting from the use of the information contained herein.

Table of Contents

INTRODUCTION 1
CHAPTER ONE 4
WHAT IS PLANT-BASED DIET 4
   8 ways to start with a plant-based diet 6
      1. Eat lots of vegetables 6
      2. Choose good fats. Fats in olive oil, olives, nuts and butter, seeds, and avocados are particularly healthy choices. 6
   BREAKFAST MEAL 7
   LUNCH MEAL 8
   DINNER MEAL 8
   WHY GO FOR PLANT-BASED DIET 8
CHAPTER TWO 17
SHOPPING LIST AND SHOPPING MENU50 TOP LIST PLAN 17
CHAPTER THREE 43
10 HERBAL BREAKFAST RECIPES TO KEEP YOU FULL ALL MORNING 43
   8. California Veggie Burger with egg on top 49
   9. Sweet Potato Breakfast 49

10. Breakfast Crunchy Salad With Eggs 50

ALL BREAKFAST FOOD 50

ALL BREAKFAST FOOD 52

CHAI SPICE RICE PUDDING (INGREDIENTS AND PREPARATION 55

VEGETABLE RICE 56

CHIA CHOCOLATE PUDDING WITH BLACKBERRY 59

HOMEMADE SOY YOGURT 61

Pumpkin Spice Cake without Gluten 63

LOW FAT CINNAMON GRANOLA.......... 65

ROASTED POTATOES WITHOUT OIL 67

HOW TO GET POTATOES WITHOUT OIL 67

BANANA CHIP ALMOND BUTTER MUFFINS 69

HASH BROWNS WITH SAUSAGE GRAVY 72

VEGAN HUEVOS RANCHEROS CASSEROLE 75

ZUCCHINI CAKES 78

HOW TO PREPARE ZUCCHINI BALL. 79

BUCKWHEAT PANCAKES 81

CORNMEAL WAFFLES 84
CHICKPEA FLOUR OMELET WITH CURRIED GREENS 86
WHOLE GRAIN MUESLI 89
SPINACH TOFU BENEDICT WITH VEGAN HOLLANDAISE......................... 91
BENEDICT WITH VEGAN HOLLANDAISE 92
VEGAN RECIPE ONLY 93
VEGETAL ADVANTAGE 93
OVERNIGHT CHIA OATS 96
CHAPTER FOUR.. 99
SOUP 99
MUSHROOM SOUP 101
Instructions 102
VEGAN CLAM CHOWDER 103
CHAPTER FIVE 107
TOMATOES BEAN SOUP 107
SAUTEED KALE SALAD 109
WARM BALSAMIC KALE SALAD 110
STRAWBERRY DANDELION SALAD 112
RAINBOW SALAD.................................. 113

REASON FOR RAINBOW SALAD 113
CHOOSE A DARK GREEN BASE 114
NUTRITION BENEFITS OF DARK GROUND AND LOSE 115
RED PURPLE VEGETABLES 115
NUTRITIONAL NAMES OF RED VEGETABLES AND PURPLE 116
ORANGE AND VEGETABLES 117
BENEFITS OF ORANGE AND YELLOW VEGETABLES 117
GREEN VEGETABLES 118
NUTRITIONAL BENEFITS OF GREEN VEGETABLES 118
WHAT ABOUT FRUIT? 119

CHAPTER SIX 121
AVOCADO SAUCE 121
Health Benefits of Avocado 121
CHEESE SAUCE 123
GARLIC SAUCE 125
HOW TO MAKE GARLIC SAUCE HOMEMADE 126

HOW TO MAKE HOMEMADE BARBEQUE SAUCE 129

CHAPTER SEVEN 131
WALNUT MILK 131
    PAPAYA SED DRESSING INGREDIENTS 136
    CUCUMBER DILL SAUCE 138
CHAPTER EIGHT 141
BREAD AND SNACKS 141
SEED CRACKERS 141
CHAPTER NINE 148
FOOD TO AVOID 148
CHAPTER TEN 160
FOOD TO CONSUME MOST 160
HEALTHFUL FOODS YOU HAVE TO KNOW 160
    Almonds 160
    Lentils 161
    HEALTH BENEFIT OF LENTILS 162
    Oatmeal 162
    Wheat germ 163
    Fruits, vegetables, and berries 164
    Broccoli 164
    Health Benefit Of Broccoli 164

- Improving bone health 166
- Improve the health of the immune system 166
- Improve skin health 167
- Promoting digestion 167
- Reduce inflammation 167
- Reduce the risk of diabetes 168
- Protection of cardiovascular health 168

Apples 169
- Neurological health and dementia 170
- Stroke 170
- Kale 171
- Health Benefit 171
- Diabetes 172
- Several nutrients in kale can support heart health. 172
- Fiber: 173
- Cancer 173
- Antioxidants 173
- Bone health 174
- Digestion: 174
- Skin and hair 174

- Eye health: 175
- Blackberries 175
- Quick facts about cranberries 175
- Health Benefit 176
- Maintaining healthy bones 176
- Skin health 177
- Reduction of blood pressure 177
- Diabetes management.......................... 178
- Protection against heart disease 178
- Cancer prevention 179
- Improving mental health 179
- Healthy digestion, weight loss and feeling full 180

- Avocado 180
  - Pineapple 181
- Green leafy vegetables 182
  - Sweet potatoes 182
  - Fish, meat and eggs............................. 182
  - Fatty fish 183
  - Chicken 183
  - Eggs.. 183
- CHAPTER ELEVEN 185

DISCIPLINE FOR GOOD HEALTH 185
IMPORTANCE OF GOOD HEALTH .. 185

INTRODUCTION

A plant-based diet may sound like vegetarianism at first, which in itself can mean a few different things. The strictest form is a vegan diet, which contains only foods from plant sources, such as fruits, vegetables, whole grains, soy products, legumes, nuts, and seeds. Many self-proclaimed vegetarians are Lacto vegetarians, meaning they eat plant foods, eggs, and dairy products such as milk, yogurt, and cheese, but not animal meat. Some consider themselves mostly vegetarian, but also eat seafood, some occasionally avoiding poultry, or perhaps simply avoiding red meat. Despite the differences, we all have in common that we focus on getting most of their nutrients from plants. Two of the most well-known plant-based diets are the Mediterranean diet and the DASH (Dietary Approaches to Stopping Hypertension) diet. Both suggest a significant increase in fruits and vegetables. Some, prefer whole grains and contain vegetable proteins such as nuts, seeds, and legumes. However, both suggest animal protein restrictions, with the Mediterranean

Diet recommending seafood over poultry and red meat being eaten sparingly. Another lesser-known but highly regarded plant-based diet in the world of food science is the Diet offers three different options for a heart-healthy plant-based diet that emphasizes more carbohydrates, proteins, or unsaturated fats, depending on an individual's preferences. Like Mediterranean and Dash, all three cartridges contain a great boost for more fruits and vegetables and the absorption of plant proteins from nuts, seeds, and legumes. It is also worth noting that all of these plant-based designs allow for dairy products in moderation all encouraging low-fat or low-fat versions and suggest limiting added sugars and refined carbohydrates.

Yes, it is technically a vegetarian diet, but there is a difference between being vegan and following a healthy vegetarian diet. The decision to go vegan comes from a person's compassion for animal life and the environment and excludes all animal products to minimize damage and inconvenience. Vegans eat a 100% plant-based diet, but not necessarily a diet based on whole, unprocessed foods. Here is the distinction.

The fundamental principle of a healthy (or "complete food") plant-based diet is to promote health and reduce the risk of lifestyle-related diseases. In addition to excluding animal products, it also excludes vegan processed products such as vegetable oils, refined carbohydrates, and foods high in refined sugar and salt.

CHAPTER ONE

WHAT IS PLANT-BASED DIET

Plant or plant nutrition patterns focus on plant-based foods. This includes fruits and vegetables, added are nuts, seeds, oils, whole grains, legumes, and beans. It does not mean that you are vegetarian or vegan and never eat meat or dairy products. Instead, divert your thinking to good things in life, such as plant-based foods. What makes plant-based diets so healthy? In addition to being low in calories and rich in fiber, vitamins, and minerals, plant foods are packed with thousands of compounds called phytonutrients ("plant" means plant in Greek) that act as natural antioxidants, anti-inflammatory and detoxifying. These compounds are mixed and blended into many combinations within plants to provide these benefits. Examples of phytonutrients are the orange-red carotenoids in carrots and tomatoes, the polyphenols in berries, tea, and dark chocolate, and the phytoestrogens in soy. Many of these compounds give plants their pigment, so the variety of colors of your fruits and vegetables and the consumption of a variety of whole grains, nuts, seeds, and legumes naturally vary these phytonutrients. What would you enjoy on a herbal-based diet? The definition of a plant-based diet may depend on who you ask. Overall, it is a diet style that emphasizes real, whole plant foods, such as Vegetables: cabbage, spinach, tomatoes, cauliflower, potatoes, pumpkin, etc. Whole grains: brown rice, oats, quinoa, barley, etc. Legumes: peas, chickpeas, lentils, peanuts, beans, etc. Vegetable proteins such as tofu or tempeh Nuts and butter Seeds

Fruit

Vegetable oils

Spices and herbs

Soft drinks: coffee, tea, carbonated water, etc.

Breakfast: oatmeal with banana slices

Lunch: black bean soup

Snack: Grilled kale with nutritious yeast

Dinner: lentil pasta with homemade tomato sauce

8 ways to start with a plant-based diet

See some points to make you started on a plant-based diet.

1. Eat lots of vegetables. fetch half of the plate with vegetables for lunch and supper. Make sure you use plenty of colors when choosing your vegetables. Enjoy vegetables as a snack with hummus, salsa, or guacamole.

Change the way you think about meat. You have smaller amounts. Use it as a garnish and not as a centerpiece.

2. Choose good fats. Fats in olive oil, olives, nuts and butter, seeds, and avocados are particularly healthy choices.

Eat a vegetarian meal once or more in a week. Make these meals around beans, whole grains, and vegetables.

Add whole grains for breakfast. Start with oatmeal, quinoa, buckwheat, or barley. Then include some nuts along with fresh fruit.

3. Go for greens. Try a variety of green leafy vegetables such as cabbage, spinach, and other vegetables every day. Steam, grill, stew or fry to preserve their flavor and nutrients

Make a meal around a salad. Fill a bowl with salad greens, such as romaine, spinach, bibb, or red leafy vegetables. Add a variety of other vegetables along with fresh herbs, beans, peas, or tofu.

4. Eat fruit for dessert. A ripe juicy peach, a refreshing piece of watermelon, or a crispy apple will satisfy your desire for a sweet bite after a meal.

Inspiration for plant-based food all-day

Over time, consuming plant-based foods will become second nature.

BREAKFAST MEAL

Oatmeal with walnuts, banana, and a pinch of cinnamon.

Wrap breakfast: Fill a wholemeal tortilla with scrambled eggs, black beans, peppers, onions, jack Monterey cheese, and a splash of hot sauce or salsa. Wholemeal English cake with slices of fresh tomato and avocado and blueberries.

LUNCH MEAL

Greek salad: chopped vegetables with fresh tomatoes, Kalamata olives, fresh parsley, crushed feta cheese, extra virgin olive oil, and balsamic vinegar. Wholemeal pie separately, fresh melon for dessert.

Tomato soup, whole meal crackers with tabouleh, and an apple.

Vegetarian pizza with mozzarella, tomatoes, broccoli, onions, peppers, and mushrooms. Fresh strawberries for dessert.

DINNER MEAL

Grilled vegetables with grilled tofu and quinoa salad and spinach. Wholemeal pasta with beans and cinnamon peas, as well as romaine salad with cherry tomatoes, topped with extra virgin olive oil and balsamic vinegar.

WHY GO FOR PLANT-BASED DIET

Plant diets are high in vegetables, whole-grain bread and cereals, legumes, and whole fruits, but may also contain small amounts of lean meat and low-fat dairy products.

1. **Reduce inflammation in your body**. If meat, dairy, and processed foods are a regular part of your diet, your body probably has a lot of inflammation. Short-term inflammation is normal and necessary, especially after a sports injury or very heavy training. However, long-term inflammation that persists for months or years is not. Chronic inflammation has been linked, among other things, to atherosclerosis, heart attacks, strokes, diabetes, and autoimmune diseases. Plant diets do just the opposite. A herbal-based diet is high in fiber, antioxidants, etc, leading to natural anti-inflammatory benefits. Fruits, vegetables, and nuts have lesser inflammatory stimuli such as saturated fats and endotoxin. This means that eating a plant-based diet can drastically reduce the levels of C-reactive protein, which is a sign of inflammation in the body. Also, animal products form incredible acids, which promotes the loss of calcium from the bones. Countries with the most beef and dairy products have the highest bone fractures. In countries where 90% of the protein comes from plant sources, on the other hand, one-

fifth of bone fractures have been reported. Unlike all advertisements, milk does not necessarily benefit the body

2. **Lower Blood Cholesterol** High blood cholesterol is a major risk factor for heart disease and stroke, two of the leading causes of death in North America. Saturated fat, which is found mainly in meat, poultry, cheese, and other animal products, contributes significantly to the level of cholesterol in our blood. Cholesterol in our food also plays a role. Studies consistently show that blood cholesterol levels are reduced by up to 35% when people go plant-based. Plant diets lower blood cholesterol as a plant-based diet, a complete diet is generally very low in saturated fat and cholesterol. Plant diets are also high in fiber, which helps to further lower blood cholesterol levels.

3. **Change the way your genes** work. Studies have shown that lifestyle and environmental factors can turn genes on and off. For example, if we eat whole plant foods, plant antioxidants and nutrients can alter gene expression to optimize the way our cells repair damaged DNA. Research has shown

that a plant-based lifestyle can lengthen our telomeres (these are the coatings at the end of our chromosomes that keep our DNA stable). This can cause our cells and tissues to age more slowly because abbreviated telomeres are associated with aging and premature death.

4. Reduce the risk of developing type 2 diabetes. It is estimated that almost 40% of Americans have pre-diabetes. Protein from animal products (especially red and processed meats) increases the risk of type 2 diabetes. Studies show that omnivores have twice as much diabetes as vegans. Even eating meat or more once a week during a 17-year study showed an increased risk of diabetes by more than 70%! Further research shows that increasing red meat consumption by more than half a serving a day equates to a 48% increased risk of diabetes over 4 years. Why does eating meat cause type 2 diabetes? Preservatives in animal fat, iron, and nitrates in meat damage pancreatic cells, worsen inflammation, cause weight gain, and reduce the action of our insulin. Non-consumption of animal products and consumption of plant-based foods will increase the chances of type 2 diabetes. Regular consumption of whole grains, which are very protective against type 2 diabetes, will promote the cause. If you already have diabetes, eating a plant-based diet can improve and even reverse type 2 diabetes.

5. A happy emotion equals a happy body. The trillions of endless microorganisms that live and form in our body are collectively referred to as the germ. Studies are increasingly showing that these microorganisms are essential for our overall health. They are important players that help us digest our food, as they produce important nutrients, help train our immune system, activate and deactivate genes, keep our gut tissue healthy and protect us from diseases such as cancer. If this is not enough, they have also been shown to play a role in obesity, diabetes, atherosclerosis, autoimmune disease, inflammatory bowel disease, and liver disease. A plant-based diet helps maintain and stimulate a healthy gut germ. The fiber in plant foods promotes the growth of healthy bacteria in our intestines. Low-fiber diets (such as high-fat dairy, egg, and meat diets), on the other hand, can promote the growth of disease-causing bacteria. When we consume choline or carnitine (found in meat, poultry, seafood, eggs, and dairy products), gut bacteria create a substance that our liver converts into a toxic product called TMAO. TMAO hosts the increase in cholesterol plaques in our blood vessels, which increases the risk of heart attack and stroke. A vegetarian meal produces little to no TMAO compared to a meal based on meat and dairy products because they have a completely different gut germ. Interestingly, it only takes a few days for the bacterial patterns in our gut to change. You will notice the benefits of a plant-based diet almost immediately. And then of course there are the large amounts of fiber, phytonutrients and antioxidants that keep the whole system cleaner. All these fibers wipe off the pathogens and keep the intestines nice and clean.

6. **Protein**- You get the right amount. Most people in North America get more than 1.5 times the recommended daily allowance of protein and most from animal sources. Contrary to popular belief, excess protein does not make us stronger and does not make us weaker. Our body can store enough protein as

fat and change into waste. Animal proteins contribute significantly to weight gain, heart disease, diabetes, and inflammation. Proteins from whole plant foods, on the other hand, protect us from many chronic diseases. Think of Popeye. He was ahead of his time and drank protein to support his active lifestyle through his favorite superfood. Spinach! As long as your daily calorie needs are met and you follow a plant-based diet, you get enough protein. Gorillas, Giraffes, Rhinos, elephants are all-powerful animals in a 100% plant diet

7. **Let your skin glow.** The easiest (and cheapest) way to have a healthy, glowing skin is to follow a clean, healthy diet without avoiding processed foods, meats, and dairy products. Your hair, eyes, skin, and nails all shine with a healthy glow from a plant-based diet. The detoxifying effect of consuming plants, the improved removal benefits and the ease with which plants are digested, all lead to less internal toxins that give us acne and more nutrients to keep our hair shiny and skin glowing. Fruits and vegetables are naturally rich in cosmetic vitamins such as vitamin C, which stimulate collagen and soften wrinkles. lycopene, which helps protect the skin from

the sun. and with antioxidants such as lutein and beta-carotene, which help soften and smooth the skin.

8. You will lose weight. Plants are generally low in calories and rich in nutrients. Calories for calories, plants give your body the greatest nutritional value for your money. Due to this nutrient density, you need less food to feel fuller. Plants are also high in fiber and keep us regular which helps us stay lean. Since plants, especially in their first form, are full of nutrients, your body has less work to do when it comes to digesting food. Because plant foods require so little digestion, nutrients are absorbed quickly, resulting in almost immediate and long-lasting energy. This abundant energy will help you exercise and stay in shape. In addition to losing a few pounds, you may also notice a drop in your cholesterol. While our genes affect our cholesterol levels, a plant-based diet can have an impact because only animal foods contain cholesterol. You do not need to tag it. Vegan, vegetables, or flexes. Whatever you call it, eating more plants is one of the deepest choices you can make. We believe that this is one of the most positive ways to live a

conscious and compassionate life. A plant-based diet will help prevent and reverse disease, significantly reduce the carbon footprint, and preserve our world for many generations. Whether you are a doctor, naturopath, paleo, vegan, omnivore or the person ordering a side of bacon with everything, we all agree that eating whole, plant foods have more nutrients, vitamins, minerals, antioxidants, fiber, and healthy fats. All of us need these things for better health. Go for the greens, spread the word, and do a little to change the world, one fork, one bite at a time.

CHAPTER TWO

SHOPPING LIST AND SHOPPING MENU50 TOP LIST PLAN

Whether you are trying to cut down on meat or become vegan, it is important to know the benefits of plant-based foods to make sure you are feeding yourself the right foods. This grocery list is your guide to including more whole foods, fun flavors, and reviewing a well-rounded meal.

1. Nutritional Yeast

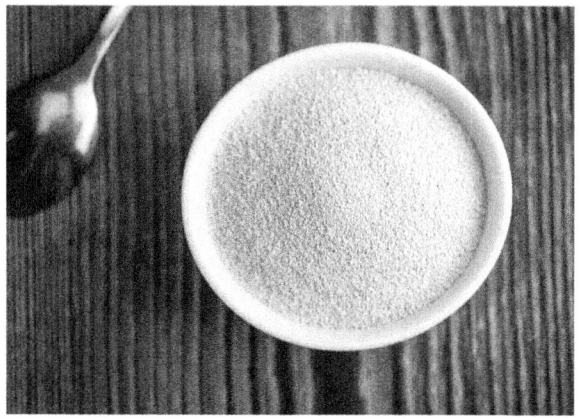

Nutritional yeast is essential for your plant-based shopping list. It is an excellent alternative to cheese because it has a similar taste and texture. Sprinkle them on your pasta, make a vegan mac n 'cheese with it, or try it on your popcorn.

2.Quinoa

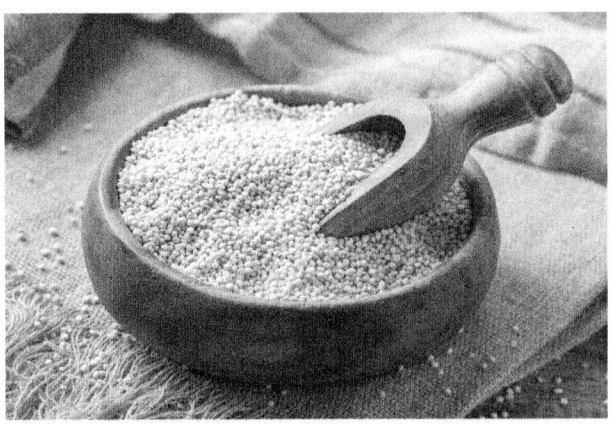

This rich source of protein contains many essential vitamins and minerals. It is an excellent base for frying vegetables. Read about ways to eat quinoa before each meal.

3.Banana

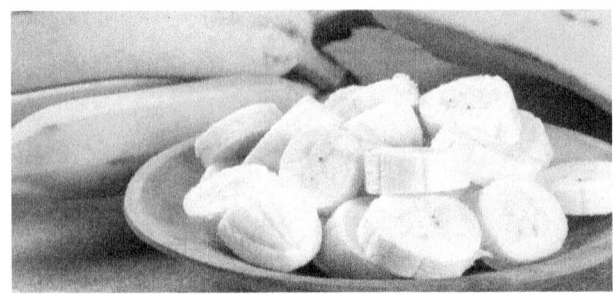

Bananas can replace an egg in cakes and pancakes. Try these Chocolate Chip banana pancakes.

4. Blackstrap Molasses

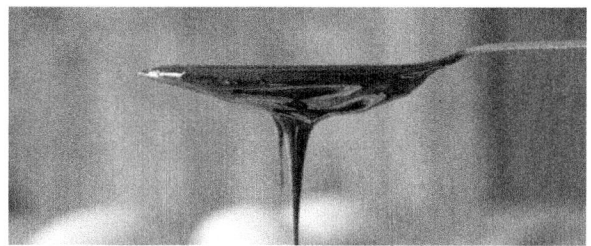

Look at the blackstrap molasses for the source of calcium without dairy products. Check out these other healthy recipe replacements.

5.Cashewseed

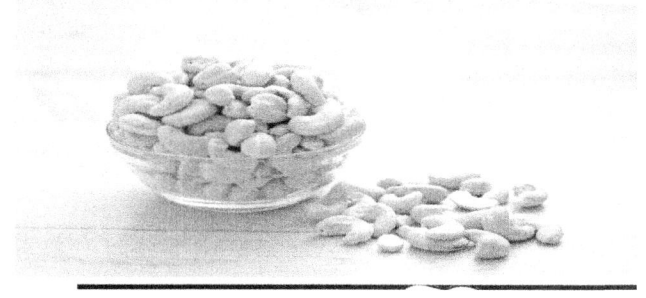

Cashews, like dietary yeast, can serve as a cheap cover for your vegan meal. Make a cashew cream with your pasta or make a raw carrot cake with cashew cream cheese. If you are looking for a healthy appetizer, try this baked pesto recipe with crispy cashew cheese.

6. **Almond**

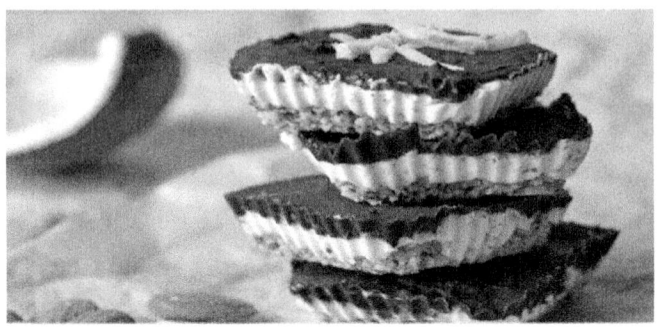

Almonds are essential for those who follow a plant-based diet because they are high in vitamin E and manganese. Take a handful as a snack or make these almond-free bars.

7. **Hummus**

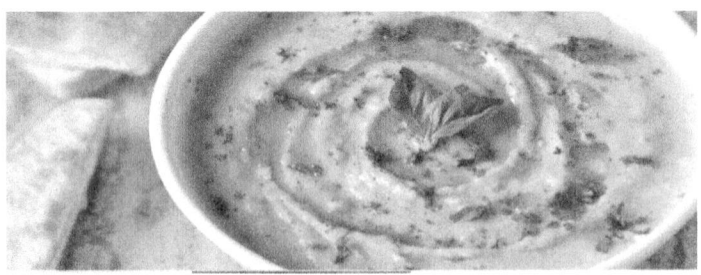

Hummus serves as a great vegan dip in addition to some chips or vegetables and can also replace your mayonnaise in a crunchy vegetarian sandwich. With each bite, you have a soft, creamy grace. Try this White Bean &

Herb Hummus.

8. Leafy Green

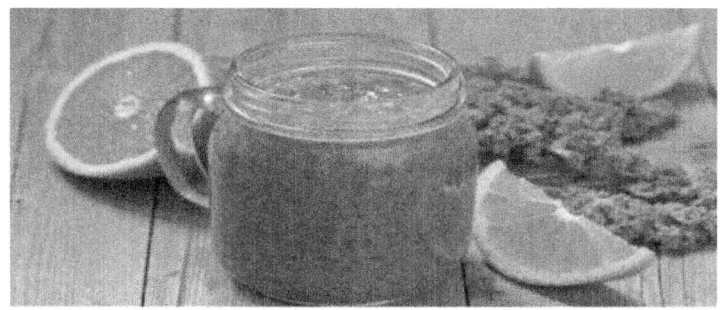

Wether it is a plant-based diet or not, leafy greens are a must. Kale is the king of superfoods, with just one cup of chopped cabbage providing levels of vitamins A, C, and K. off the chart. Start your morning well with this good and smoothie.

9. Edamame

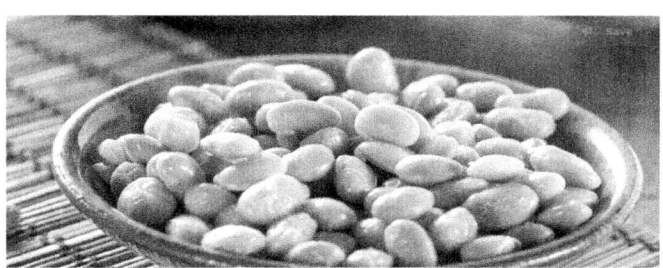

Getting enough protein when cutting or screwing meat may seem impossible, but this is because plant-based protein choices are less commonly advertised. One cup of soybean has as much as 17 grams of protein. Edamame is a super clean eating snack, like these other Clean Eating Low-Calorie Snacks.

10fronzenfruit

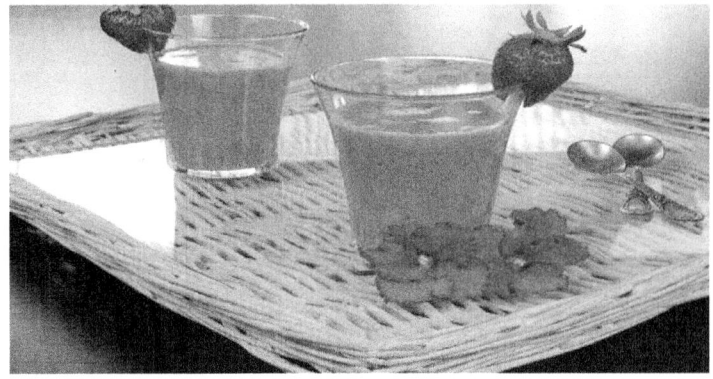

Budget-frozen fruits are a great addition to your list of plant-based nutritional requirements. Full of vitamins and antioxidants, frozen fruit can be used regardless of the season. Berries are brain foods, so add them to your smoothie, like this vegan Quinoa, Banana, Berry Smoothie.

11. Organic Sprouted Grain Bread

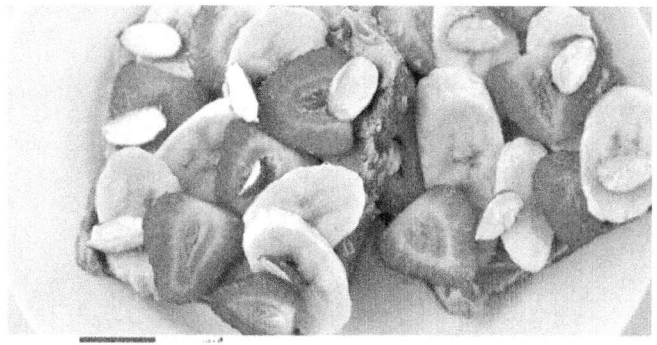

Did you know that some types of milk contain ingredients? Choose bread with organic plants to avoid the risk of dairy products! Make this and place it on top of the sprouted bread. Make this whole wheat peanut butter & fruit toast with sprouted bread.

12. Seaweed

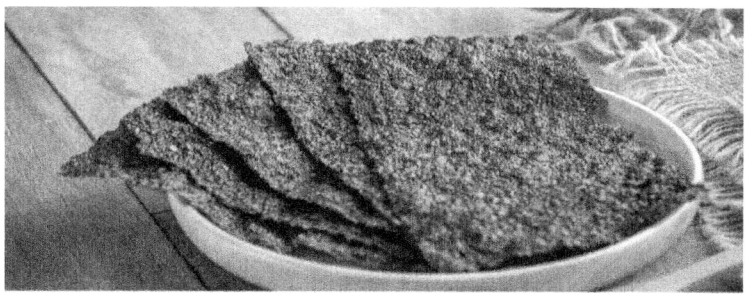

Rich in omega-3 fatty acids, seaweed is a must for vegans. Plus, it's another excuse to order this exciting seaweed salad during the sushi night! Check out these 3 wonderful seaweed snacks for your healthy body.

13. Dry Lentils

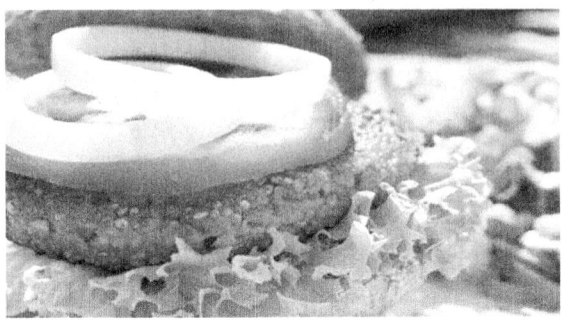

Lentils provide 16 grams of fiber and 18 grams of protein in a single cup. If you like a big juicy burger, try this Quinoa Lentil burger!

14. Tempeh

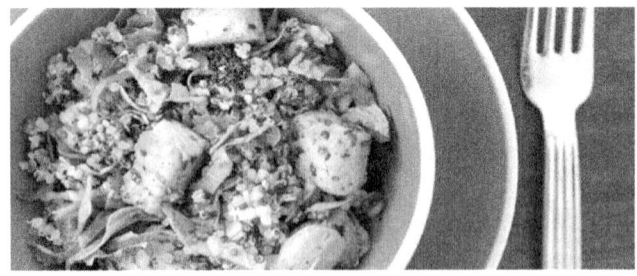

This fermented soy product has a wonderful nutty taste and chewy texture, making it extremely versatile for your protein needs. This maple Tempe glass with quinoa and cabbage is unique, clean, and delicious.

15. **Coconut Oil**

If you need butter for cooking or baking, replace it with respectable coconut oil. See 6 reasons later why you should eat a tablespoon of coconut oil daily.

16. **Avocado**

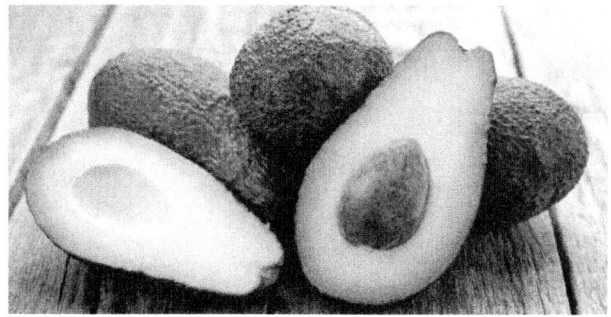

Avocados provide the creamy texture you want in dairy products, as well as healthy fats and fiber, vitamin B6, potassium, protein, and magnesium. Add avocado to your dessert with this Vegan Fudge Brownie avocado recipe.

17. Cauliflower

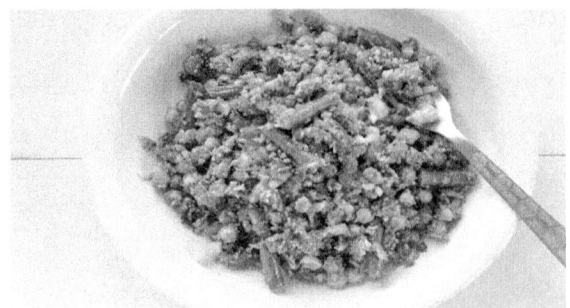

Cauliflower is such a versatile vegetable cross. Make it on your pizza crust, puree it, or use it as the main ingredient in a curry dish. Make a healthy Chinese dish with this Super Easy Fried Rice Cauliflower.

18. Squash

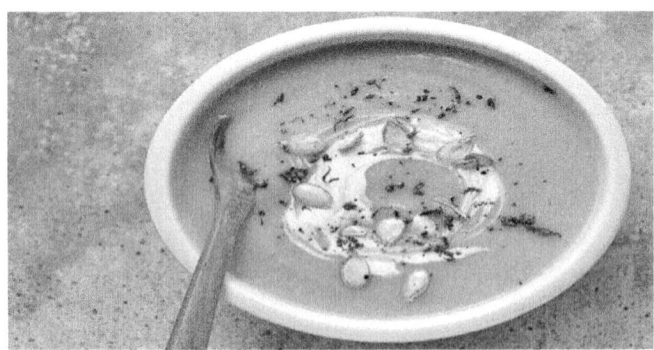

More like a vegetable, this fruit can be prepared in many ways. It is a filling option with omega-3 fatty acids, B vitamins, iron, and potassium. If you like soup, this Slow Cooker Carrot Squash soup is a must!

19. Carrots

Get vitamin C, A, beta carotene, and fiber carrot fixation. Enjoy raw, steamed, grilled, or grilled! These Carrot Spice oatmeal cookies are a vegan delight

20 Beets

The beets have a great taste, while their color can enliven a dish. Try this unique Blood Red Beet Hummus with carrot fingers for a healthy and fun aperitif.

21. Artichokes

Artichokes are a nice addition to your grocery list with plant foods and full of spicy flavor and add to a bowl of vegetables. They are also high in protein and contain 4 grams in half a cup.

22. Asparagus

Asparagus adds a deep green hue and rich flavor to meals, and also contains 4 grams of protein per cup, as well as vitamin B6, potassium, and folic acid. If you like a bowl of vegetables, try this roasted asparagus and pepper recipe.

23. **Mushrooms**

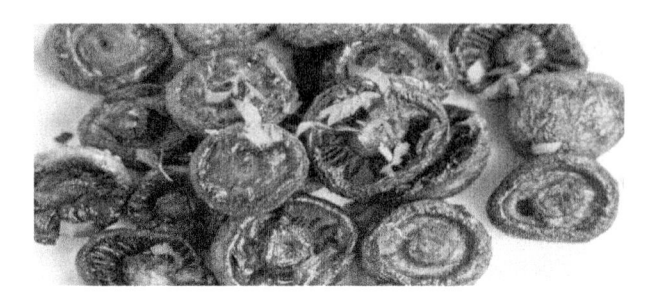

The fleshy texture of the mushrooms and the higher humidity during cooking are an excellent alternative to meat. There is so much flavor, just eat it, as in this toasted mushroom clean food is sure to curb your craving for a bite of beef

24.**Oats**

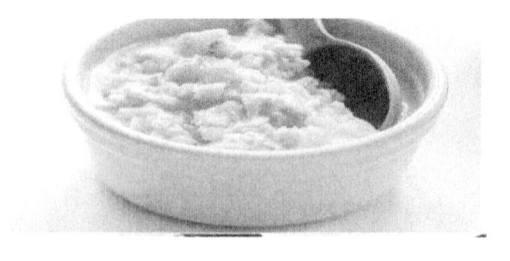

Fill up on oats in the morning to get a healthy dose of protein so you feel energized and satisfied throughout the morning.

25. Amaranth

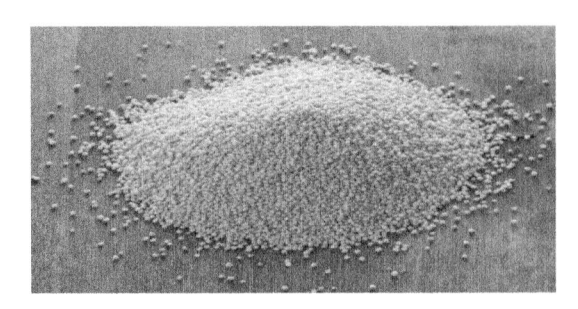

Perhaps a lesser-known grain, amaranth offers a sweet and savory taste. It is also packaged with protein and provides 6 grams per cup. Some of these 7 clean breakfast portions of cereal contain amaranth.

26. Buckwheat

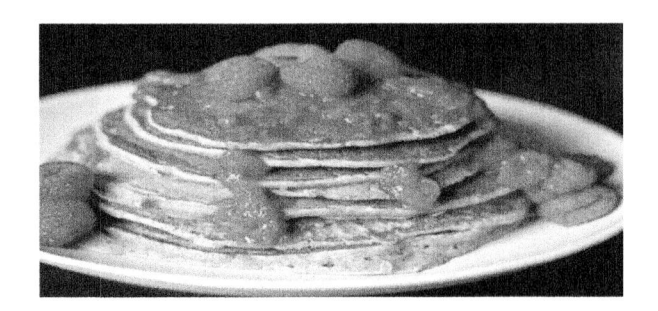

Use buckwheat flour if you have a gluten intolerance. It will give you the protein and magnesium you need for energy and vitality. These Strawberry Rhubarb Buckwheat Bars will make you swoon.

27. Teff

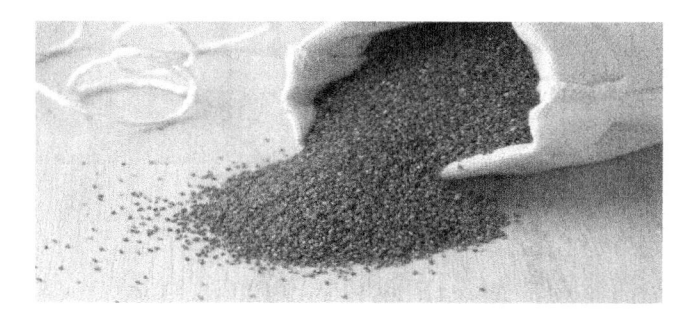

Teff may be small in size, but it has a huge protein content, at 7 grams per 1/4 cup. It's great for a gluten-free diet.

28. Flax, Chia, and Hemp Seeds

These tiny seeds are packed with omega-3 fats, iron, magnesium, and fiber. Add them to your breakfast, sprinkle them with a salad, or bake them on your cookies. Change your breakfast with this Mango Chia Breakfast Bowl.

29. Sunflower Seeds

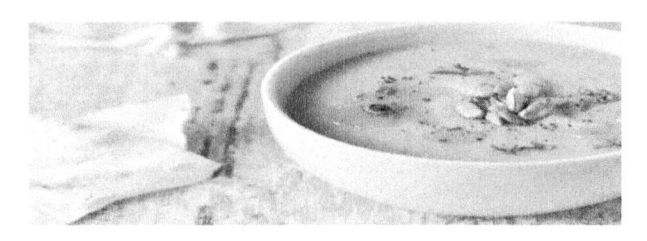

Rich in vitamin E, sunflower seeds are a great snack for more energy and focus. Sunflower Lentil Dip is highly recommended.

30. Walnuts

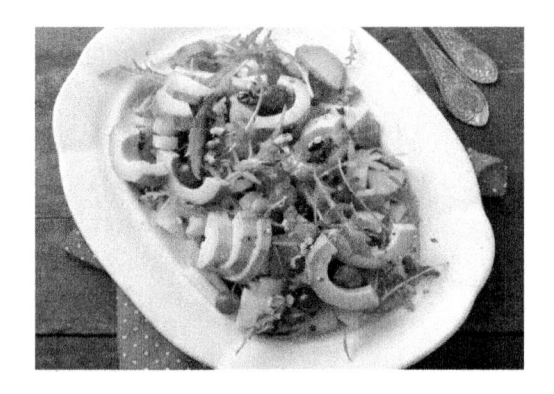

Walnuts are an excellent source of vitamin E, magnesium, and omega-3 fats. You can even grind them to replace meat in tacos. Add a little crunchy to your salad with this avocado and grape salad with walnuts.

31. Soy Milk

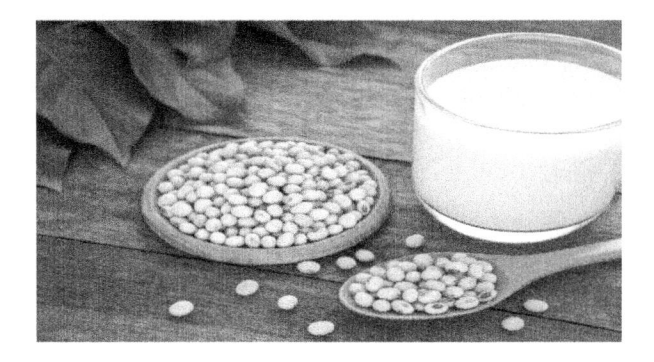

Replace the cream in your coffee or milk in your breakfast cereal with soy milk, which provides about 7 grams of protein per cup. Is a Yummy Dairy Free Milkshakes.

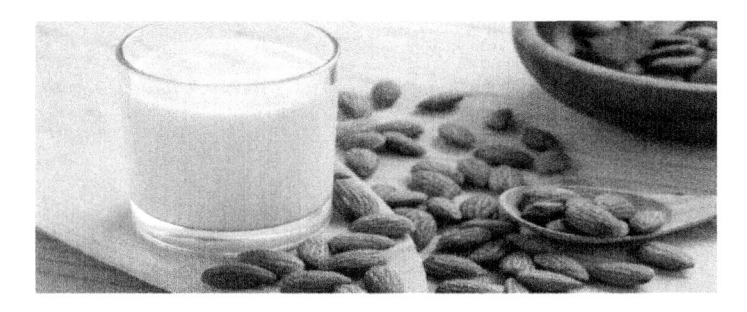

32. Almond milk

Almond milk, which contains heart-healthy fats, is another great alternative to regular milk. Try using it in cream-based recipes. Read later the process of producing milk alternatives here.

33. Coconut Milk

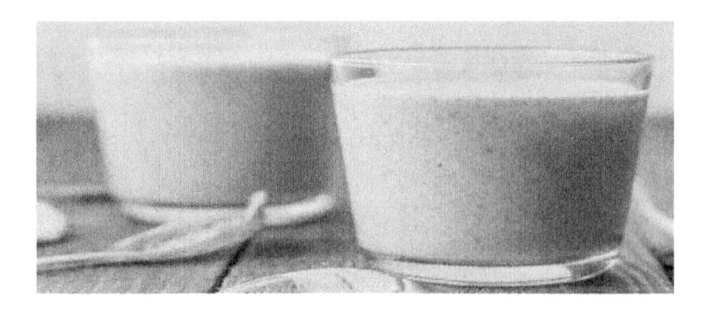

Did you know that coconut milk contains 50% more calcium than dairy milk? It is wonderful coffee milk, in addition to smoothies, and gives a wonderful taste to baked goods. This coconut milk smoothie is so delicious.

34. Cashew Milk

If you like the taste of cashews, add sweet and creamy cashew milk to the shopping list based on your plant-based diet.

35. Rice Milk

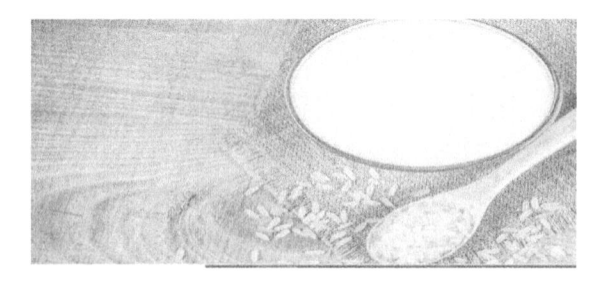

In addition to being non-allergenic, rice milk is low in fat and high in niacin, vitamin B-6, iron, copper, and magnesium. Make your milk with this cinnamon rice milk recipe.

36. Oat Milk

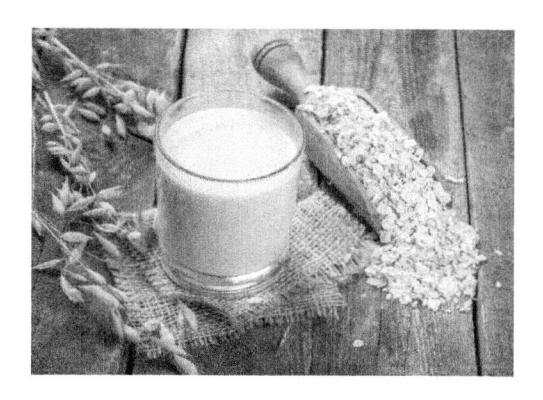

A relatively new milk alternative on the market, oat milk provides fiber and protein, at about 4 grams per serving.

37. Hemp Milk

This complete protein provides you with a recommended daily intake of omega-3 fats in a single serving! Swap almond milk and replace it with hemp milk in this Protein Smoothie.

38. Aquafaba

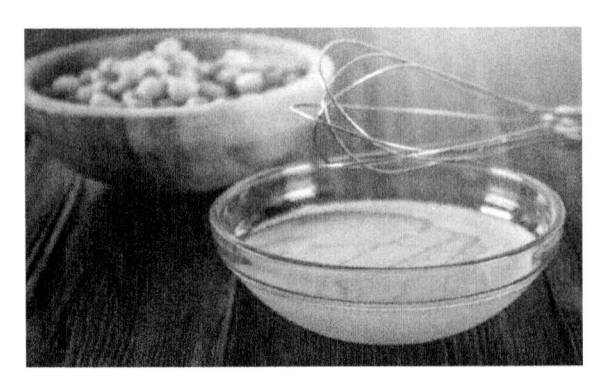

Do you shrug your shoulders with this? It may not sound familiar, but we'd love to hear it first! It is the high-starch liquid found in a can of cooked chickpeas and serves as a thickening and foaming agent. It is a great alternative to eggs, with one tablespoon of aquafaba equal to one egg yolk and two tablespoons equal to one egg white. Be sure to save the chickpea juice when you make this baked sweet potato recipe stuffed with hot curry and chickpeas!

39. Seitan

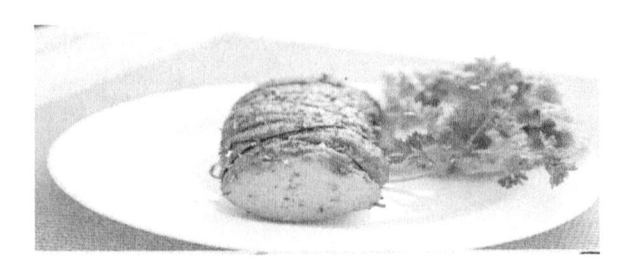

If you can handle gluten, add seitan to your plant-based diet list. Gives a chewy texture and works well with a variety of spices. It is full of protein, without cholesterol, and extremely versatile.

40. Sweet potato

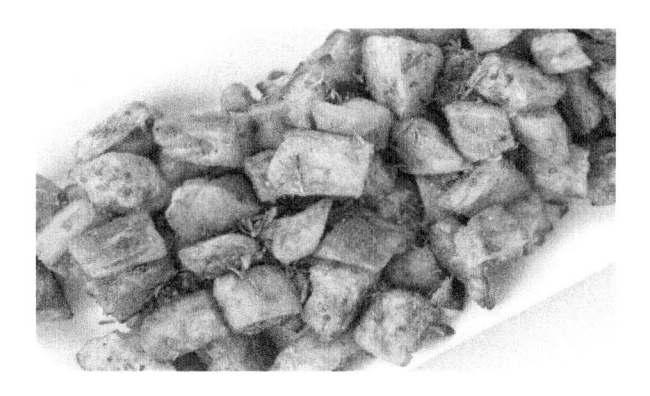

Sweet potatoes are a super-food full of beta carotene that fights cancer. Get out of the box of a simple baked potato and try this roasted sweet potato with turmeric and cardamom recipe.

41. Veggie sausages

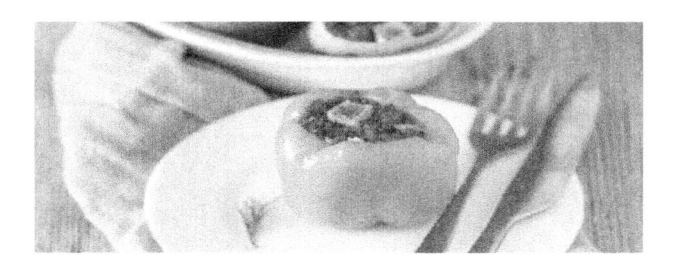

Fake meat can be packaged with processed ingredients. To avoid this, choose a brand that offers good things, such as Field Roast. Replace turkey sausage with vegetable sausage and vegetable broth with chicken to enjoy this recipe for stuffed peppers with fennel and sausage as a vegetable meal

42.Veggie burgers

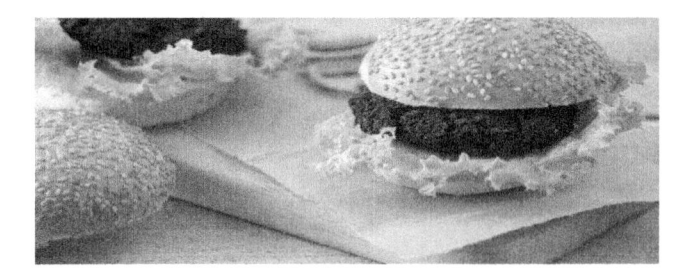

Vegetable burgers are so easy to make and so delicious

43. Soy yogurt

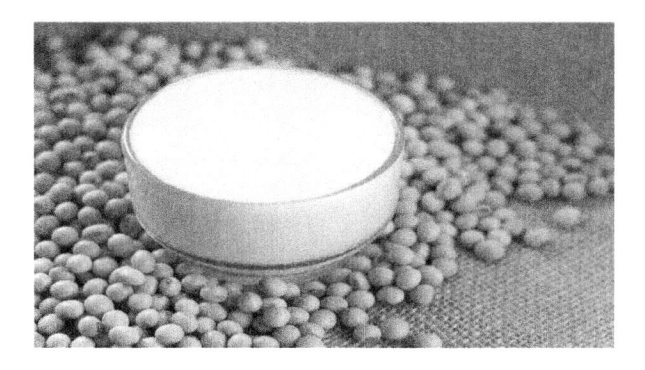

Give your emotion a little love soy yogurt snack. It is full of probiotics! Try the cool cucumber soup with rose petals used in soy yogurt in this article covering the yin and yang of cooking.

44. Agar

This vegan gelatin substitute is perfect for creating vegan jello! Try this garbage-free Jello.

45. Miso paste

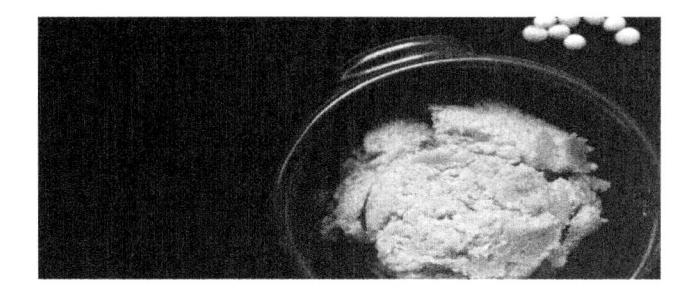

Who says plant foods should be mild? Miso paste is a great addition to the list of plant-based groceries, as it adds umami to vegetables and serves as an excellent anchovy substitute. If you like miso, try this miso outfit.

46. Vegetable broth

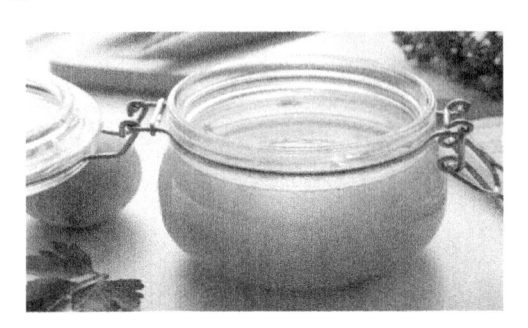

So many recipes require broth and it adds so much flavor instead of water when cooking quinoa. Try this Cilantro Lime three bean salad with vegetable broth.

47.Tomato paste

Tomato paste is a rich source of iron. Add it to your lentil stew for a red hue and an added touch of flavor. Learn how to make this Homemade Canned Tomato Paste.

48.Sun-dried tomatoes

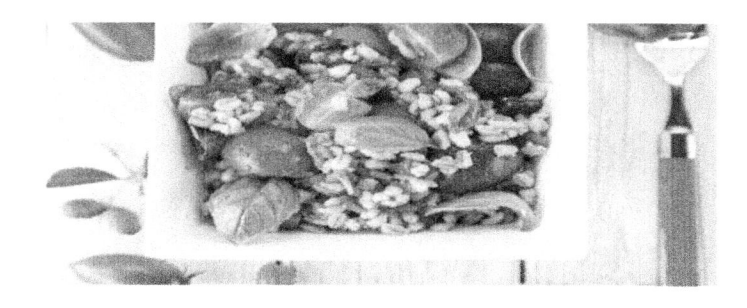

Fantastic for adding texture and flavor. Try this colorful, satisfying, and delicious Barley with Fresh and Sun-Dried Tomatoes recipe.

49. **Capers**

Capers are a savory, delicious addition to your meals. Try this delicious lemon Vinaigrette.

50. **Tahini**

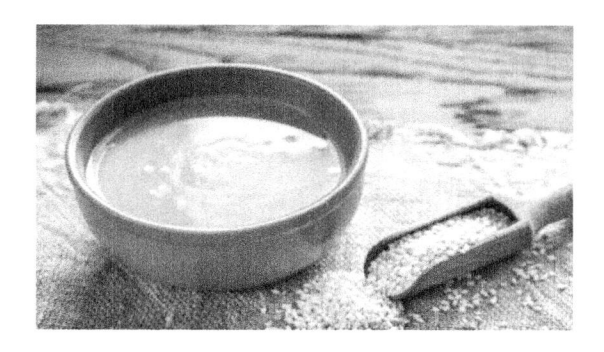

Tahini or sesame paste, is an excellent vegetable spice that is rich in minerals such as phosphorus, lecithin, magnesium, potassium, and iron. Try this homemade baked falafel with spicy Tahini sauce. There are so many delicious ways to start your plant-based diet and these simple, savory, sweet, unique choices prove it!

CHAPTER THREE

10 HERBAL BREAKFAST RECIPES TO KEEP YOU FULL ALL MORNING

Breakfast is a very important meal it can either make or break your day, so why not add some vegetables to your plate?

Say goodbye to boring breakfast and say hello to a meal that will keep you going until lunch. While Passerby may have probably promised you a mild breakfast many times before, they have probably not been as healthy, as convenient and as delicious as these plant-based breakfast recipes. Whether you are on a vegetarian diet or just want to eat more plants, there is no better place to start with breakfast. These recipes take advantage of the saturating properties of plants to make your day successful. Bookmark this page as you try each of these plant-based breakfast recipes.

1. **Wholemeal vegetable pancakes with cashew butter** wholemeal pancake on a vegetable basis

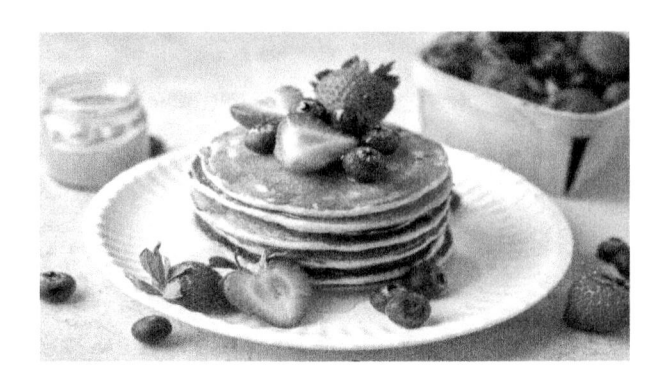

This recipe for vegetable pancakes proves that you can follow a plant-based diet and enjoy your favorite foods. In this recipe, we use a mixture of protein-rich pancake and waffle mix with hemp milk, and on top with cashew butter and fresh fruit. Eating a protein-rich breakfast like this will keep you full all morning you will never go back to the old box mix after that. Get our recipe for wholemeal vegetable pancakes with cashew butter.

2. **Vegetable lentils and kale**

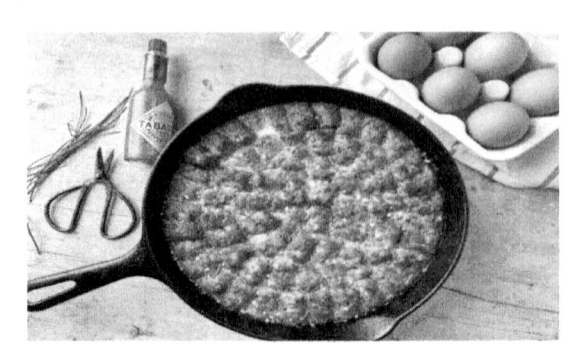

Are you looking for an easy way to include more vegetables in your diet? Replace your shoes with this good one. (Do not worry, they still have potatoes!) Combine these leafy green toddlers with fiber-rich lentils, seasoned with the same spices found in the average breakfast sausage. Even better than this herbal breakfast recipe that helps you eat more vegetables for breakfast could be the fact that you can make this pot in advance and throw it in the oven the next morning.

3. Black Bean & Vegan Sausage Grain-Free Burrito

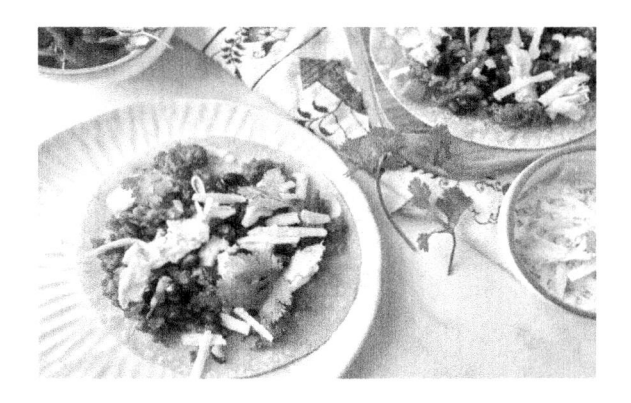

While your typical breakfast burrito may be high in fat and sodium, this vegetable burrito uses a mixture of ground vegetables such as meat, black beans, and eggs. And before you think you are losing protein by switching from chorizo to vegetable, think again. The reasons we use Light life contain 20 grams of protein per serving. This plant-based breakfast recipe is perfect for brunch on Sunday or even as a meal. Simply wrap each burrito in foil, freeze and seal in an airtight container. To warm, remove the foil, cover with a damp paper towel, and microwave until well warmed.

4. Avocado Crispbread with all Bagel herbs

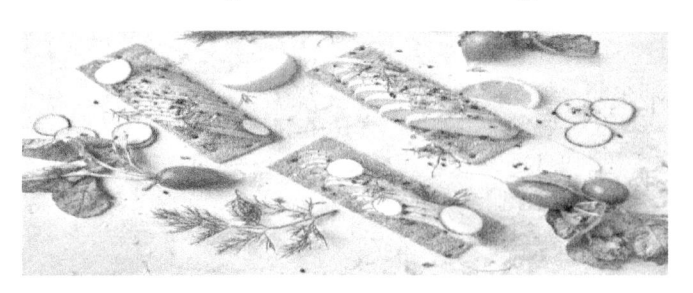

For a lighter version of avocado toast, replace your high-carb bread with Finnish wholegrain rye chips one of our favorite healthy crackers. We like to fill our creamy avocado with fresh lemon, dill, radish slices, and all the spices for a great taste that is still calorie-conscious. If you are looking for a high protein breakfast, add lox! Salmon is rich in omega-3 fatty acids that can help reduce the risk of cardiovascular disease.

5. Breakfast Burrata Dippers

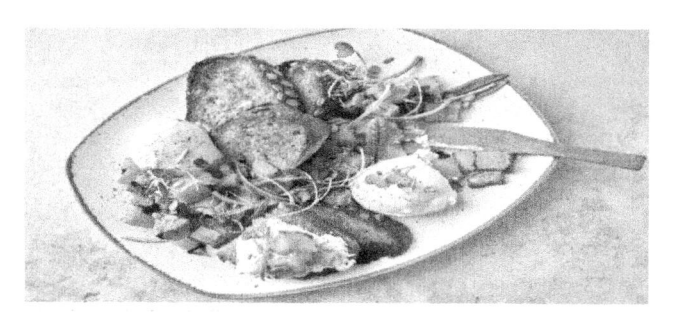

Inviting people to a brunch? Did you keep a burrata from a meat platter from last night? Do you just want a creamy, rich, nutty and caramelized breakfast? There is nothing better than this bowl of burrata breakfast. But get ready for squash and burrata your family will ask for seconds after the first bite.

6. Vegan Sausage Sheet Pan Veggies

You can find these vegetables and vegan sausages traditionally in an omelet, but you do not need eggs here. Not only will you save yourself the hassle of cleaning multiple pots and pans, but you will also have a clean, plant-based breakfast.

7. Vegan Mediterranean tofu

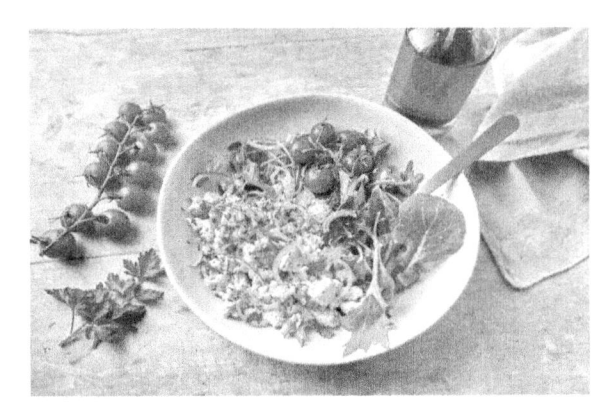

If you love eggs but are looking for a plant-based alternative, try tofu! To make this eggless game, you will want to catch solid or very hard varieties of tofu. Season the protein-rich tofu with red pepper, feta, parsley, and tomato to incorporate Mediterranean flavors. Looking for extra flavor? Try sun-dried tomatoes in oil, capers, or even olives.

8. California Veggie Burger with egg on top

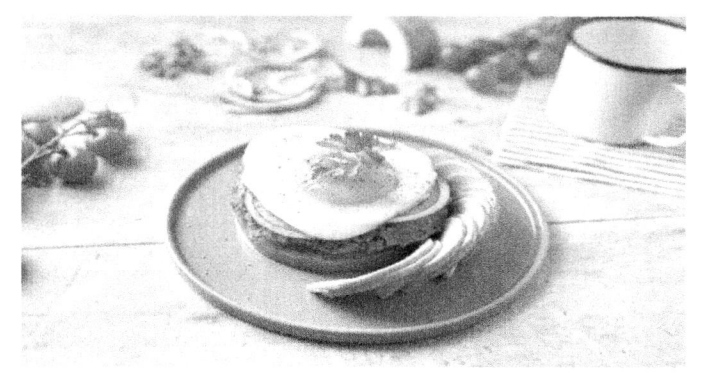

If you are tired of yogurt at work, we have another simple breakfast idea for you. Store some vegetarian burgers in your office freezer. Put it in the microwave and you can go. We chose to go without bread using a rich slice of tomato and adding onions and avocado. When you are at home, fry a wet egg. At work? Bring some soft boiled eggs to serve on top.

9. Sweet Potato Breakfast

Did you bake the sweet potatoes last night? Do you go grain-free or gluten-free? This breakfast is for you. This vegetarian breakfast is a variation on the traditional baked potato, replacing sour cream with protein-rich Icelandic yogurt. Top with crispy granola and sweet blueberries. You can eat the whole sweet potato rich in fiber skin and stuff but be sure to rub the skin before baking.

10. Breakfast Crunchy Salad With Eggs

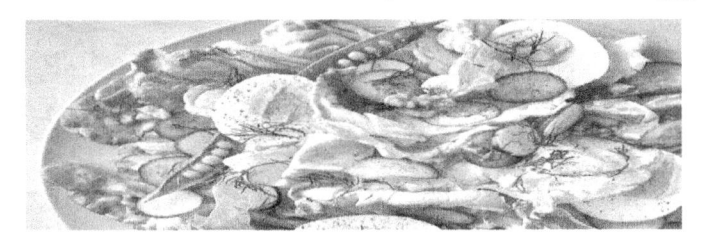

Have you ever been sick of a sweet breakfast? Contrary to popular belief, you do not need to swallow 20 grams of sugar during your breakfast. Sprinkle the lettuce you planned for lunch and cook some eggs. (Just make sure you use the strict boiled egg technique.) Top up with a spicy balsamic sauce for a delicious, herbal breakfast recipe to eat over and over again.

ALL BREAKFAST FOOD

A plant-based breakfast is a great way to start your day. And, a great time to get some of your portions of fruit with smoothie or oatmeal with berries. It is easy to forget about fruit for the rest of the day, so if you need 5-7 servings a day, start right away. Most plant-based breakfasts are easy to make, such as oats that are ready to eat at night if you are in a hurry in the morning.

ALL BREAKFAST FOOD

Super Seed Chocolate Oatmeal

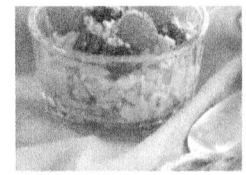

Chai Spice Rice Pudding

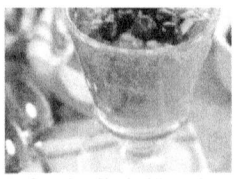

Chocolate Chia Pudding with Blueberries

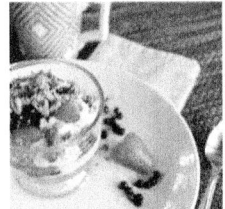

Homemade Soy Yogurt

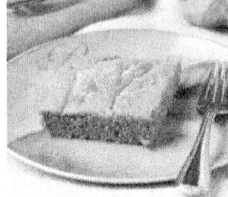

Gluten-Free Pumpkin Spice Cake

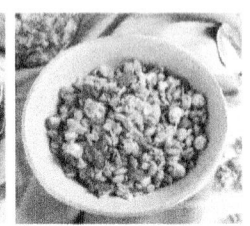

Low Fat Cinnamon Nut Granola

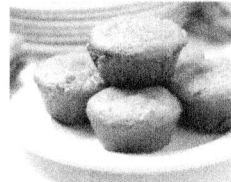

Banana Chip Almond Butter Muffins

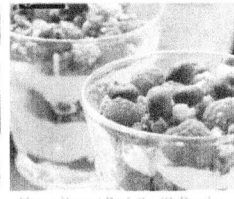

Vegan Yogurt Parfait with Berries & Granola

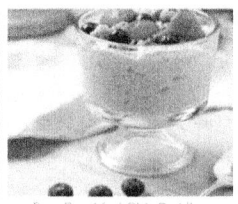

Easy Breakfast Chia Pudding

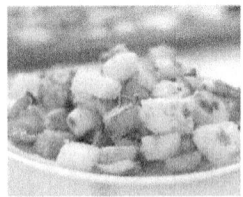

Oil-Free Roasted Potatoes

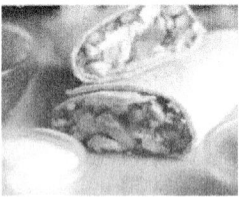

Breakfast Burrito with Tofu Scramble

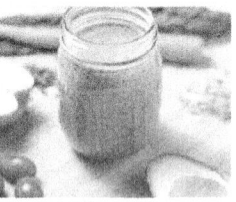

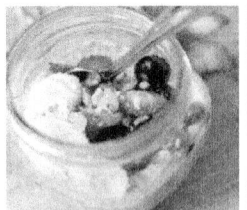

V 8 Smoothie

Overnight Chia Oats

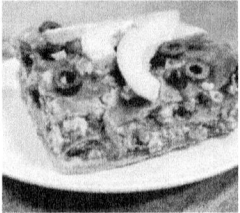

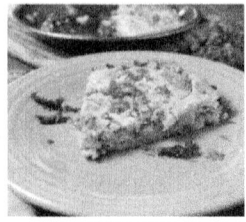

Vegan Huevos Rancheros Casserole

Crustless Broccoli Sun-Dried Tomato Quiche

53

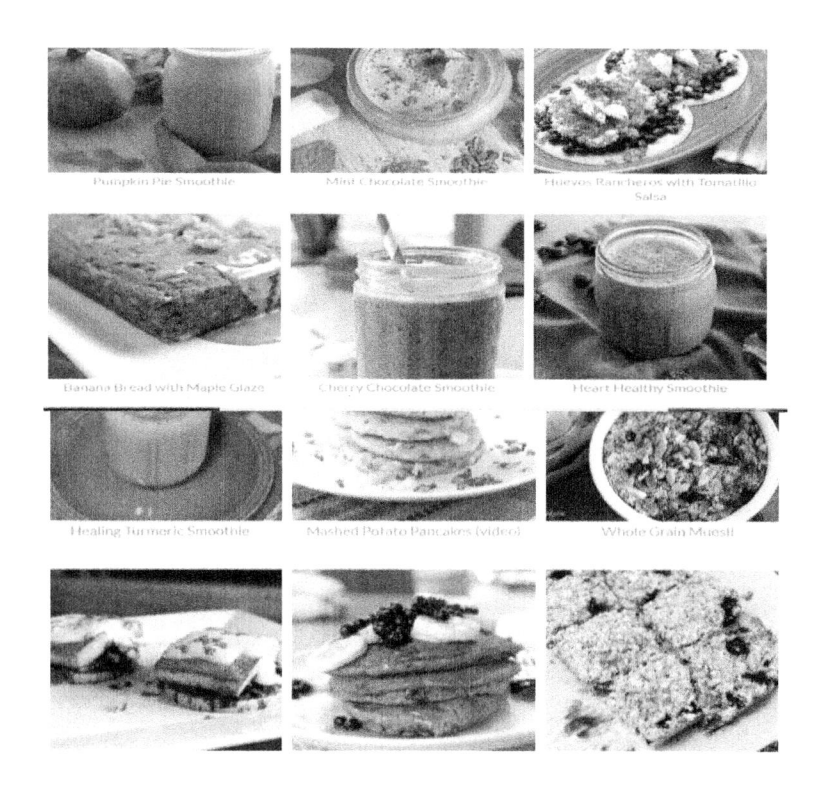

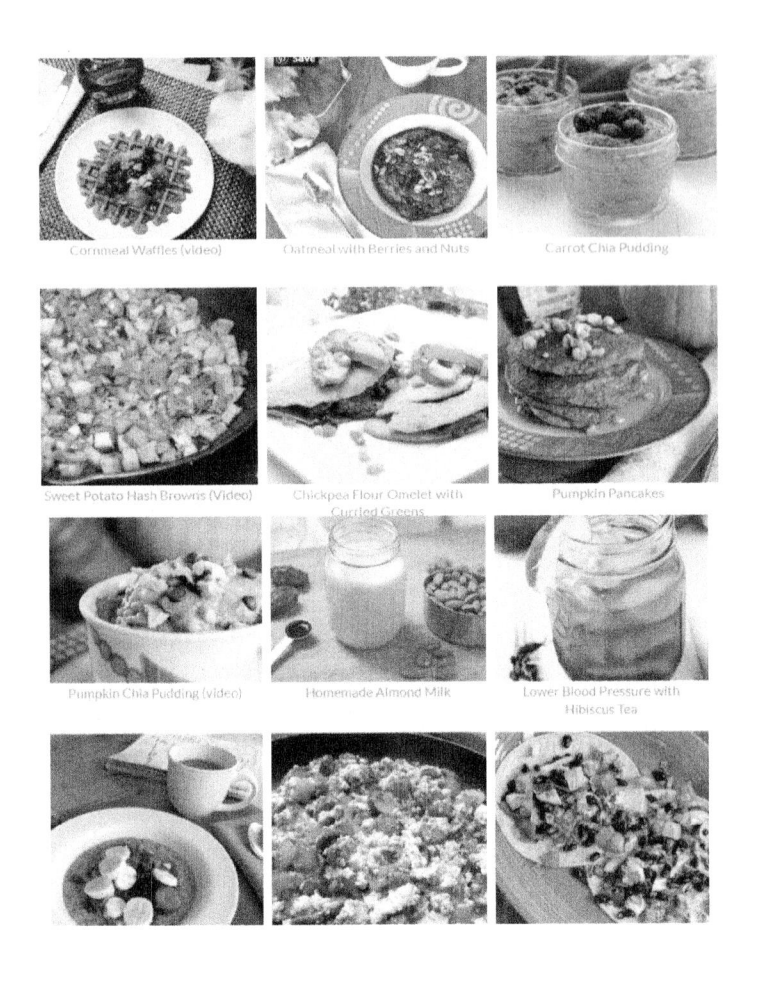

Cornmeal Waffles (video) — Oatmeal with Berries and Nuts — Carrot Chia Pudding

Sweet Potato Hash Browns (Video) — Chickpea Flour Omelet with Curried Greens — Pumpkin Pancakes

Pumpkin Chia Pudding (video) — Homemade Almond Milk — Lower Blood Pressure with Hibiscus Tea

CHAI SPICE RICE PUDDING (INGREDIENTS AND PREPARATION)

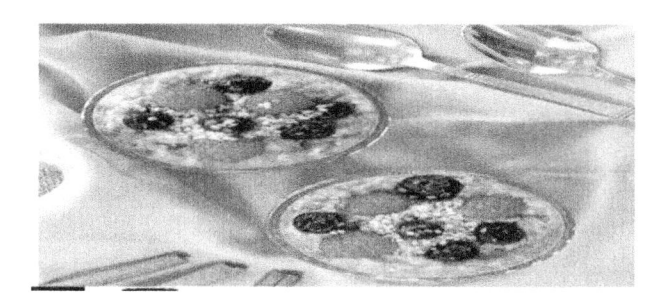

Rice pudding is a creamy, soothing dessert that is also great for breakfast or snacks. You can easily make it from scratch with non-dairy milk of your choice. I like to use soy milk because it adds more protein than other vegetable milk. Try the sugar-free Eden Soy for more protein and cream.

Rice pudding, raspberries, blackberries

Coconut milk is another popular choice, but it is not recommended for a plant-based diet because it contains little saturated fat. If you stay with rice, this is great for this rice pudding recipe.

VEGETABLE RICE

When preparing the rice, I make sure to rinse it well under running water, because in case you have not heard it yet, the rice contains some traces of arsenic. Take a look at my article "The Low-Down on Arsenic in Rice" if you want more information. Then put all the ingredients in the pan and cook until the rice is cooked. Be careful because I have noticed that the rice tends to swell on the lid and sometimes overflows. Stirring will sometimes prevent this. Rice pudding If you are not a fan of chai spices, you can skip the cardamom and spice and it will be just as good. And you can choose your favorite sweetener or sugar substitute. The recipe uses maple syrup, but coconut or sugar from the date works like date syrup. The toppings make this dessert special. I like to finish it with fresh berries and nuts, but you can choose your favorites. What about banana or mango or spicy yogurt? ince this recipe is made with brown rice and chai spices, it has a warmer color than white rice. I like to make rice pudding from scratch because the creamy milk is poured into the rice, but if you already have rice left, you can do it as follows.

Add 2 cups remaining rice to a pan over medium heat. Add 1 + 1/2 cup milk, vanilla, spices, and sweetener and cook, uncovered, for about 20 minutes until the pudding thickens. Stir regularly. When the rice starts to dry, add up to 1/2 cup of milk

Chai Spice rice pudding

This vegan chai spice rice pudding is a creamy, soothing dessert that is also great for breakfast or snacks. Use your favorite vegetable milk and sweetener.

Preparation time 5 minutes

Cooking time 45 minutes

Portions

Components

1 cup brown jasmine rice

2 cups non-dairy milk (any type will do)

1 cup of water

1 teaspoon vanilla extract

1 teaspoon of Ceylon cinnamon

1/2 teaspoon cardamom

1/2 teaspoon allspice

1/4 cup maple syrup

Top options

2 tablespoons hemp

1 cup berries

1/4 cup chopped walnuts

1/2 cup yogurt without dairy

Rice pudding, raspberries, blackberries

Instructions

Rinse the rice with running water and put it in a medium saucepan. Add non-dairy milk, water, spices, and vanilla. Cover and heat until boiling. Lower and cover. Cook for 45 minutes or until rice is cooked There may be excess liquid, but rice should absorb it as it cools.

Watch the pan and stir regularly because the rice tends to swell on the sides of the pan. Drain the excess water after the rice has softened. Add more sweetener if you want a little sweeter.

Serve sprinkled with a garnish of your choice.

CHIA CHOCOLATE PUDDING WITH BLACKBERRY

Chia seeds are a quick and healthy way to thicken recipes because they are unique in that they swell dramatically and form a gel syrup called tapioca. They can be used to make a simple jam, toss smoothies, put oats in the evening, and, most of all, make chia pudding like this chocolate Chia pudding with blueberries. They are also full of healthy goodness because they contain omega 3 fatty acids, are high in fiber, and even contain proteins and minerals. While chia seeds are both lighter and almost black, it does not matter who you use in a recipe, unless you want to keep the color consistent, as, in a lighter pudding, you may want to use lighter chia seeds.

Chocolate Chia Pudding-2 Chia seeds take about two hours to swell enough to thicken pudding, so plan if you want to serve it for dinner. For this recipe, all you have to do is add the seeds to your favorite vegetable milk, along with the flavors and pudding, cool in individual serving dishes, or a larger bowl. For it to cool, put in the fridge.

Chia chocolate pudding with blueberries

This wonderfully simple recipe is perfect for both company and a delicious breakfast. Chia seeds stand out quickly in the fridge and are ready at any time of the day.

Preparation time 10 minutes

Components

2 cups non-dairy milk without sugar

1/3 cup chia seeds

1/4 cup cocoa powder (or cocoa powder)

1 teaspoon vanilla extract

1/4 cup maple syrup (or more if you prefer it sweeter)

1 box of fresh or frozen blueberries

1/4 cup sliced almond

Chia-2 chocolate pudding

Instructions

In a medium bowl, combine cocoa powder, vanilla extract, maple syrup, and vanilla with a little vegetable milk until smooth. Then add the remaining milk. Stir to combine. Try and if you want sweeter, add more maple syrup or Stevia.

Add the chia seeds and mix. Cool for a few hours until the chia seeds swell, stirring occasionally to mix.

If the mixture looks like pudding, put it in individual serving dishes and fill with blueberries or another of your favorite fruits and some grated almonds or leave it in the bowl and refrigerator for 4-5 days.

HOMEMADE SOY YOGURT

If you think yogurt production is out because you do not have a yogurt maker, guess what you can still make yogurt! Here are to grow yogurt without making yogurt.

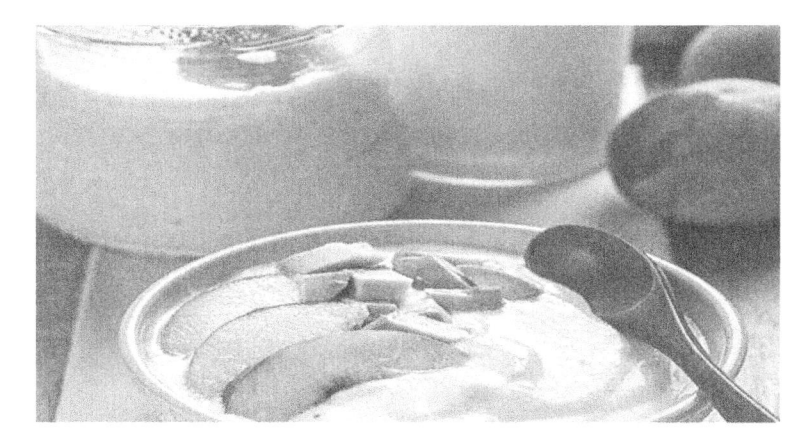

Homemade soy yogurt

Now you can make your delicious soy yogurt in your kitchen. It becomes nice and thick. Add a little sweetness or add fresh fruit when it is ready for a delicious addition to your breakfast.

Preparation time 25 minutes

Components

3 Tbl of corn

1 32 ounces soy-free milk without sugar

1-2 Tbl maple syrup

1 yogurt starter pack

Soy yogurt breakfast

Instructions

Add 2 cups of soy milk to a saucepan and begin to heat over medium heat. Be careful when heating, as it can boil over the edge of the pan if you do not look at it or heat it too quickly.

Pour 1/2 cup cold soy milk into a measuring cup and beat at 3 Tbl. corn.

Once the milk starts to steam, whisk the cornstarch lightly. Continue to heat to 148 degrees and beat until slightly thickened.

Remove from heat. Beat the remaining soy milk and let the temperature drop to at least 110 degrees

Beat in the starter to mix and pour into your container (s).

Pumpkin Spice Cake without Gluten

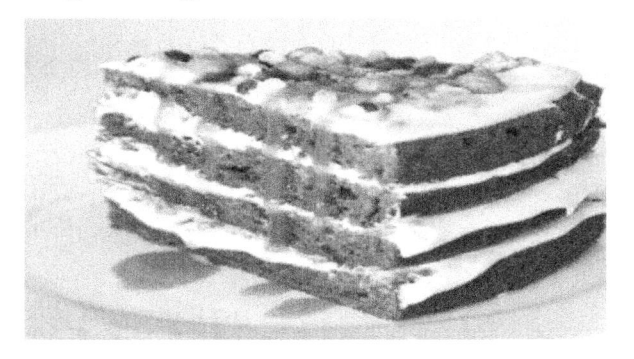

Components

Liquid materials

3/4 cup pumpkin puree (or sweet potato puree)

1/4 cup non-dairy milk

1 teaspoon vanilla

1/3 cup maple syrup

2 teaspoons apple cider vinegar

1/4 cup date sugar, erythritol sugar substitute or date sugar (optional for more sweetness)

Dry ingredients

1 cup all-purpose gluten-free flour (I used Bob's Red Mill with a combination of beans and GF flour)

1/2 cup almond flour

1 Tbl pumpkin spice

2 tablespoons

1/3 teaspoon sea salt

Pumpkin spice cake-2

Instructions

Preheat the oven to 350 ° F (180C). Line a 20 x 20 cm baking tray with baking paper. Tip: crumble the baking paper first and then smooth it out. It forms much easier on the saucer. Or spray lightly with cooking spray.

Using a whisk, mix all the liquid ingredients in a bowl until combined.

Mix the dry ingredients in a second bowl and add to the liquid ingredients. Stir until mixed.

Spread the batter evenly on the baking tray.

Bake for 30 minutes or until a toothpick or a sharp knife comes out. It. may take some minutes, depending on the oven.

LOW FAT CINNAMON GRANOLA

You will not believe how easy this homemade low-fat granola recipe is from scratch and it does not take much time to make. Enjoy a few spoonful's of your favorite yogurt or mix it with fresh fruit.

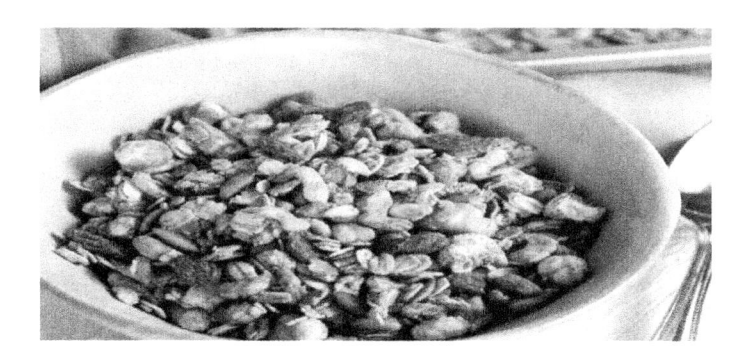

Components

2 cups whole oats

2 cups popped corn

2 cups puffed millet

1/2 cup sliced almonds, walnuts or peanuts

3/4 cup dried blueberries without sugar

1/2 cup apple sauce without sugar

1/4 cup date syrup or maple syrup

1 drop full of liquid sweetener Stevia (optional)

2 teaspoons Ceylon cinnamon

1 teaspoon of non-alcoholic vanilla extract is preferred

sea salt excursion

1/2 cup grated coconut (optional)

Instructions

Preheat the oven to 300 degrees.

Measure the oats, corn, and millet in a large bowl and add the walnuts.

In a separate small bowl, add apple sauce, maple syrup, cinnamon, vanilla and sea salt and mix well.

Add liquid ingredients to breakfast cereals and mix to combine.

Spread on two baking sheets covered with parchment.

Bake every 15 minutes for 30-45 minutes until lightly browned.

Add dried fruit (and grated coconut if using) and mix.

ROASTED POTATOES WITHOUT OIL

Oil-free baked potatoes are a perfect dish if you are looking for recipes based on whole foods.

Since potatoes remain on the menu, I'm looking for ways to use them without added fat. I like to steam instead of boiling because it retains more of the nutrient content of the potato instead of rinsing it in water.

HOW TO GET POTATOES WITHOUT OIL

Can you roast potatoes without oil? The trick with these oil-free roast potatoes is to boil them a little so that they cook a little. Then put some flour in the pan after draining, cover, and shake like crazy! Now your potatoes should be crushed a little and sprinkled with flour. This is one of the secrets to making potatoes crispy and for these oil-free baked potatoes.

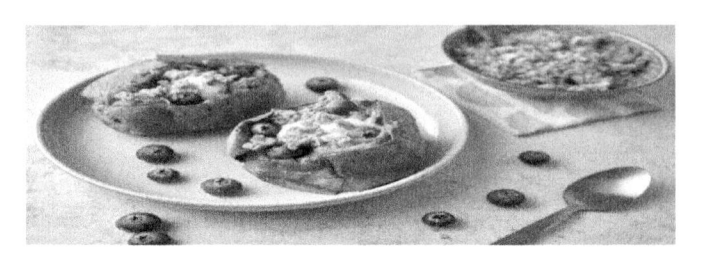

Components

2 large russet potatoes, peeled and cut into 1 piece.

2 large yams, peeled and cut into 1 piece.

1 large pepper in each color, cut into 1 pumpkin pieces

1 large red onion cut into 1 cut pieces

2-3 Tbl wholemeal flour

Baked potatoes without oil

Instructions

Preheat the oven to 450 degrees F.

Put the potatoes, onion, and peppers in a large pan with a little water and when the water boils, steam for about 5 minutes until the potatoes are crisp.

Drain the vegetables, but leave them in the pan (do not put the pot back on the fire) and sprinkle the flour on it.

Place the lid back on the jar and shake vigorously for a few seconds. Destroy the edges, which will later facilitate the crunch of the potatoes.

Discard the potatoes in olive oil or use parchment paper or silicone and make sure they are in a layer (do not stuff the potatoes or the edges will not become crispy). Sprinkle with salt and pepper.

Bake at 450 degrees F for 30-45 minutes, turn after the middle, but be careful not to burn.

BANANA CHIP ALMOND BUTTER MUFFINS

Warm and soothing with a touch of sweetness and wholemeal, this Muffins Butter Banana Chip Almond Butter is a delicious dessert that is healthy enough for breakfast. Once you make a batch, breakfast becomes a breeze.

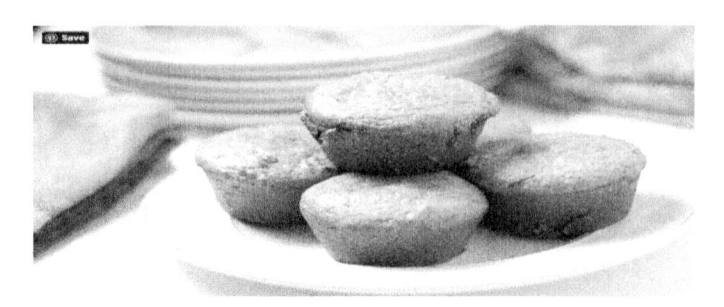

Start with banana and almond butter with a touch of maple syrup and coconut or date. Optionally add non-dairy chocolate chips and or chopped nuts and you're almost there.

Components

1 cup ripe banana puree

1 cup almond butter

4 Tbl maple syrup

2 teaspoons vanilla extract, non-alcoholic, preferably

4 Tbl date sugar or coconut sugar

2 flax egg 3 Tbl water + 1 Tbl ground flaxseed

1/2 teaspoon sea salt

1 teaspoon baking powder

1 teaspoon baking soda

2/3 cup oatmeal + 1 tbsp

2/3 cup oatmeal

2/3 cup non-dairy mini chips (optional)

2/3 cup chopped walnuts (optional)

Instructions

Preheat the oven to 350 º F

Injection of 12 large muffin cans (not paper bags) with non-stick coating

Beat by hand or with banana, almond butter, honey, vanilla, and sugar in combination. Add the flax eggs.

Combine dry ingredients, oatmeal, salt, baking soda, baking soda, and salt. Add the liquid ingredients and mix to combine.

Mix the oats and the mini chips (the mixture will be sticky).

Fill muffin tins with batter.

Bake at 350 º F for 15-18 minutes

Try with a toothpick. When dry, they are ready.

HASH BROWNS WITH SAUSAGE GRAVY

You need to make some elbow fat for Easy Gravy, but it's a quick recipe. When you have collected all the ingredients, wholemeal flour, yeast, Tamari onion powder (or soy sauce), vegetable stocks and some non-dairy milk, just put them in the pan and mix.

If you like the sauce on the white side, skip the vegetable and add only non-dairy milk. If you want your sausage to brown, you can brown it in a separate pan.

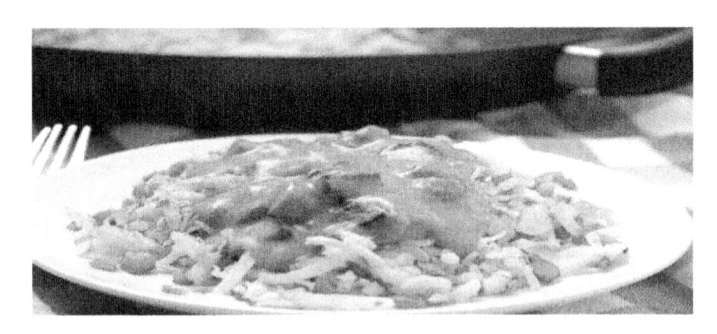

COMPONENTS

Easy sauce

1/3 pound vegan breakfast sausage cut into small pieces

3 Tbl whole wheat or unground flour

1/2 teaspoon onion powder

2 Tbl nutritious yeast

1 cup of homemade

1 cup non-dairy milk

2 tablespoons tamari or soy

Sea salt and pepper

Grated french fries

1 pound frozen brown gold without added oil

1/2 onion cut into cubes

1 pepper of any color, stems, without seeds and cut into pieces

2 cloves garlic, minced meat

Remove 1 small Jalapeño seeds and veins, thin slices (optional)

Chives for garnish

Country Hash with sauce

Instructions

Easy sauce

Cook the vegan sausage in a medium non-stick pan over medium heat until golden brown. Sprinkle the sausage with the onion powder, the nourishing yeast, the salt, and the pepper on top of the sausage.

Add the vegetable, non-dairy milk, and tamarind or soy sauce and mix lightly. Continue stirring on the stove until the broth starts to thicken. Reduce heat and keep warm.

Grated fresh fries

Heat a large non-stick pan over medium heat. Separate the frozen brown herbs from the pan and cook for 6-10 minutes, then turn and cook for another 5 minutes, until golden brown.

Add the chopped onion, garlic, and pepper and mix to combine. Flatten the potatoes and vegetables evenly again and let them sit until golden brown again. You can keep turning and browning the brown until it is as crisp as you want.

Serve fragmentation sprinkled with breakfast sauce and topped with chives.

VEGAN HUEVOS RANCHEROS CASSEROLE

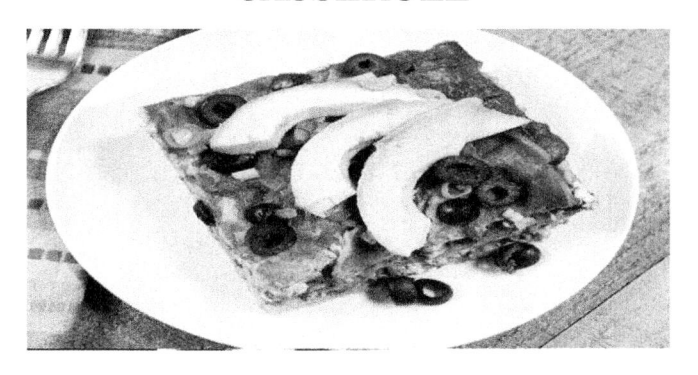

COMPONENTS

1 pack of corn tortillas (8 measurements)

2 15 ounces. cans of black beans (without salt) drained, rinsed and lightly mashed with a fork (Eden Brand) (or 3 cups homemade)

1 Jalapeño without seeds and thin slices (optional)

2 large avocados cut in half and sliced

1/2 6 ounces can drain the low salt black olives and cut them

Easy Ranchero sauce

½ large yellow onion cut into cubes

1 clove of garlic cut into cubes

1 Jalapeño without seeds and in cubes (optional)

1 teaspoon Ancho chili powder

1 box of organic tomatoes 14.5 ounces (without added salt, Muir Glen brand)

1 14.5 ounces can fry roasted tomatoes (without added salt, Muir Glen brand)

2 cups low-sodium vegetable broth

1/4 cup chopped coriander

Tofu Scramble

1 12-14 ounces drained heavy organic tofu

1/3 cup diced onion

1/3 teaspoon turmeric

sea salt and pepper

Instructions

Tofu Scramble

Preheat the oven to 350 ° F.

Fry the chopped onions in a medium saucepan in a little translucent water and usually cooked.

Grate the curd and add it to the pan for color together with the turmeric. Stir to combine and continue cooking until most of the water has evaporated and the ingredients are cooked through.

Easy Ranchero sauce

In a large saucepan over medium heat, fry the onion and pepper in a little water. Allow the water to evaporate and brown the vegetables slightly. Season with salt and pepper.

Add the rest of the sauce ingredients, lower the temperature and simmer uncovered until slightly thickened, about 30 minutes.

When the sauce has thickened a little, remove from the heat and let it cool a bit. Be careful when mixing a hot sauce as it may splash if it is too hot, but at this point mix the sauce ingredients until soft. A food processor must also work.

Spoon a small amount of rancher sauce on the bottom of the pan and spread with the back of a spoon. Fill with a layer of tortilla, separate to fill the pan, and fill with a little more sauce.

Place 1/2 of the black beans on the tortillas.

Top with 1/2 of the tofu scramble, ranchero sauce and then another layer of tortilla.

Tortillas with rancher sauce, beans, stir, sauce, and a layer of tortilla.

Finish with sauce to cover the tortillas so that they do not become too crisp in the oven.

Seal with foil and cook in the oven for about 30 minutes. Locate and check for liquid in the pan. If there is a little, put it back in the oven for about 5 minutes.

Serve with sliced olives, green onions. optional jalapenos and avocado slices

ZUCCHINI CAKES
Easy Beans Zucchini

Simple ingredients, quick to prepare, and easy to prepare, this zucchini cake recipe is a delicate and delicious dish for any occasion.

Recipes often require squeezing the zucchini to get rid of water after rubbing, but with the addition of flour, it is not necessary. Vegetable water helps to make the batter.

Adding chickpeas to this recipe boosts your vegetable protein and is an excellent egg substitute. They are also rich in nutrients and offer many health benefits such as weight management, lowering blood sugar, and digestion. These will be healthy zucchini cakes. If you are not a fan of onions or just want to add a little color and extra vegetables, add a little grated carrot.

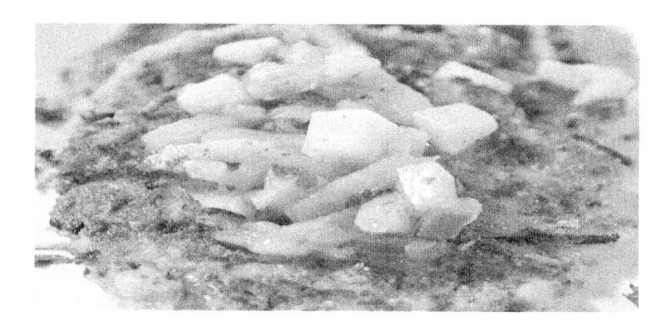

HOW TO PREPARE ZUCCHINI BALL

Combine zucchini, chickpeas, and red onion in a bowl. Then dry the ingredients and the flax mixture, salt (optional), and mix until well mixed. Each cake is about 2-3 tablespoons and this recipe should produce about 8 cakes.

Try a spoonful of mango salsa, a spoonful of yogurt, or even a splash of maple syrup with fresh lemon pressed on it to add an extra touch of flavor to these zucchini cakes.

Components

1 Tbl ground flaxseed and 3 Tbl water

2 medium grated zucchini

1/3 15 ounces can puree chickpeas (or use a food processor, but keep a few larger pieces)

2 Tbl red onion grated

1/4 cup corn

3 tablespoons flour

1 teaspoon baking powder

1/2 teaspoon sea salt

homemade mango salsa

Instructions

Combine the flaxseed meal and 3 Tbl of water in a small bowl and let it rest for about 10 minutes.

Include chickpeas, red onion, and zucchini to a bowl.

Add the corn oil, flour, baking powder, flax mixture, and salt. Stir until well combined.

Spray the pan with cooking spray and add about 2-3 T of the mixture, leveling.

Cook each side for about 2 minutes.

Serve with chutney or mango salsa and possibly add a dash of lemon.

BUCKWHEAT PANCAKES

Can't get enough pancakes? There are so many versions but these buckwheat pancakes are naturally gluten-free because buckwheat is not a cereal and does not contain gluten.

Buckwheat is a seed that is rich in fiber and protein. With oats added, you have a heart-healthy dynamite pancake.

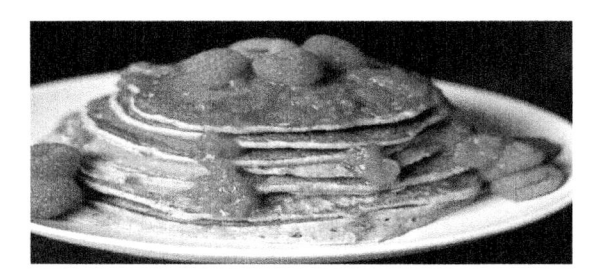

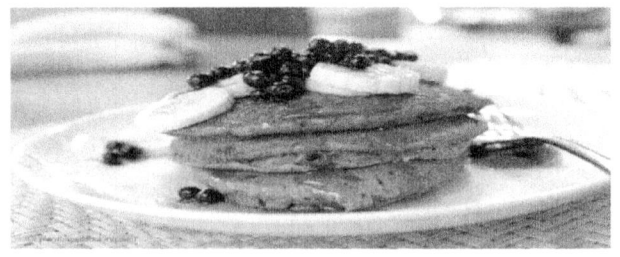

INGREDIENTS

1 cup buckwheat flour

1/2 cup cornmeal

1/2 cup old-fashioned or instant oatmeal works

1 teaspoon baking soda

1 teaspoon baking powder

1/4 teaspoon sea salt or to taste

1 teaspoon Ceylon Cinnamon

1-1 1/2 cups non-dairy milk

1 large banana, frozen or fresh

1/2 cup apple sauce

1 teaspoon of the best non-alcoholic vanilla extract

1 tablespoon optional maple syrup

1/2 cup chopped walnuts or mixed nuts

1 cup frozen or fresh blueberries

Instructions

Combine all dry ingredients, from buckwheat to cinnamon.

If you use a fresh, ripe banana, make it first with a fork and a bowl. Mix it with the rest of the wet ingredients, from non-dairy milk to maple syrup. Thaw frozen banana in the microwave first.

Put the wet ingredients on the dry and stir until it mixed. Let stand for a minute. Add a little more non-dairy milk if it is too thick.

Heat a nonstick skillet (add a little oil spray to a metal skillet if you use it) and drop about 2 large spoonfuls into the pan. Turn up when the edges appear dry.

Do not overestimate. This can lead to drought.

Place on a plate and serve with blueberries, banana slices, maple syrup (or more apple sauce), and nuts.

CORNMEAL WAFFLES

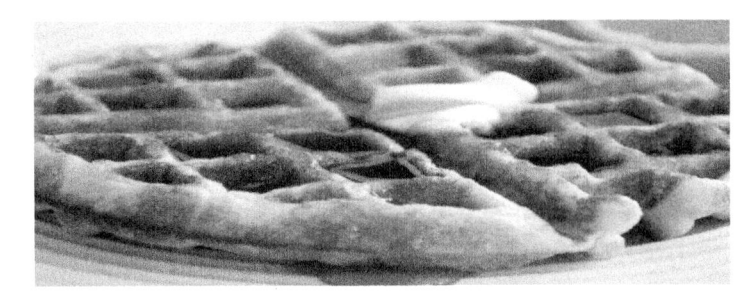

Ingredients

1 cup cornmeal

½ Cup of Oats

2/3 cup whole white flour

½ Teaspoon Baking soda

½ teaspoon of sea salt

1 teaspoon of ground cinnamon

½ Cup of almond or soy milk or other breast milk

1/3 cup apple sauce

1 tablespoon maple syrup

1 tablespoon optional coconut oil

½ teaspoons prefer non-alcoholic vanilla extract

1 cup Blueberries

Maple syrup

2/3 Cup Garlic

Instructions

Combine wet ingredients, milk, apple juice, maple syrup, and vanilla extract in a bowl.

In another bowl, combine the dry ingredients, cornmeal, oats, flour, baking powder, salt, and cinnamon.

Add the dry ingredients to the liquid and mix thoroughly.

Bake in your waffle according to the instructions.

To make the blueberry syrup, take a little maple syrup over the cup of blueberries and heat for a few seconds in the microwave.

Top each waffle with a spoonful of apple juice, blueberry maple syrup mixture, and a few nuts.

For gluten-free use 1/3 cup buckwheat flour

CHICKPEA FLOUR OMELET WITH CURRIED GREENS

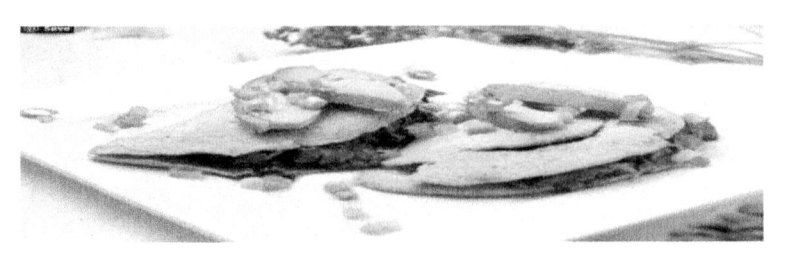

Looking for a great egg substitute for your omelets?

Try the Chickpea Flour! Because chickpeas or garbanzo beans, if you prefer have a good amount of protein 6 grams per 1/4 cup of flour. One egg is just over 6 grams.

This omelet looks more like a pancake and it can be a little cozy, so most recipes pump it up with spices and herbs.

You can add all sorts of ingredients to chickpea flour omelet dough - chopped basil or spinach, sun-dried tomatoes, and green onions or roasted peppers. However, if you have a hearty oven like this Chickpea Flour Omelet with Greens, a more neutral aroma will be a nice contrast.

I have used spinach in this recipe, but you can use kale or Swiss skewers. Sometimes kale can be chewy unless it is cooked long enough, so I find spinach to work better. Falafel recipes often use chickpea flour in connection to chickpeas.

Ingredients

1 pack spinach or kale chard.

1-2 cups prepared spaghetti sauce I like Whole Foods 365 Fat-Free Organic Brand Pasta Sauce.

1/2 teaspoon of curry powder

Add salt and pepper to taste

I used 1 cup of Chickpea flour from Bob's Red Mill brand.

1/4 teaspoon baking powder

1/2 teaspoon ground turmeric

1 tablespoon dried herbs such as parsley, marjoram

2 tbl nutrition inheritance optional

1/2 teaspoon sea salt (or to taste)

1 cup water and more if needed

Sliced.avocado for garnish

4 green onions, cut

Chickpea Omelet

Instructions

Cut charcoal spinach, cabbage, or kale and put them in a large frying pan with about 1/2 cup of water.

Sauté until tender

Add 1 to 2 cups of pasta sauces and curry powder to the pan and continue to cook until heated through and the green vegetables are dead. Include some water to thick.

Combine the cherry flour, baking powder, dried turmeric, nutritional herbs, dried herbs or seasonings, and salt and pepper.

Add the water and lemon juice and stir to combine the ingredients. It should be the consistency of a pancake batter, edible and not too thick. Adding more water is needed to get the right consistency.

Heat your pan over medium-low heat. If you are using a non-stick pan, the omelet should come loose if you have cooked it long enough. Otherwise, use a small metal dish and touch it with cooking spray. Remember, you must not use cooking spray on non-casserole dishes.

Pour 1 / 4-1 / 3 cup of dough into the pan and rotate to move the dough to the edges. If it is too thick, use a spatula to help you. The top of the omelet will look like a cake button and brown on the ground. You can put a lid on the oven to help cook the oven. Wait until it is slightly brown to "free" it from the pan with your spatula. If it looks like it's cooked enough, you do not need to transform it.

Using your spatula, fry the omelet and place it on a plate.

Using a large spoon, place 1/4 of the curry filling on one half of the omelet and fold the other half over. Garnish with avocado slices.

WHOLE GRAIN MUESLI

This recipe includes oats, white flakes, quinoa flakes, hemp hearts, ground flaxseeds, almonds, pumpkin seeds, nuts, coconut flakes, and raisins. A blend of whole grains, without added oil, nutrients, nuts, and seeds for a vegan herb stock.

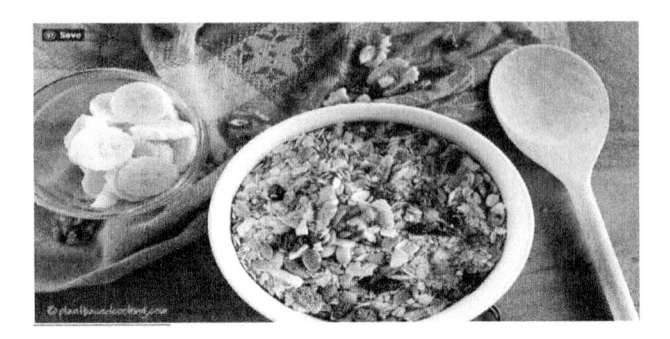

Ingredients

2 cups of old-fashioned oats

1 Cup Uncle Sam Brand White Flakes

1 cup quinoa flakes found next to the warm cereal

1/2 cup hemp hearts

1/2 cup Ground Flax Seeds

1/2 cup sliced almonds or sliced whole almonds

1/2 cup raw pumpkin seeds

1/2 cup nuts

1/2 cup coconut flakes

1/2 cup raisins or other raisins do not contain sugar

1 teaspoon Ceylon Cinnamon

1 teaspoon almond extract

Instructions

Put all ingredients in a large bowl and mix to combine.

Store in a glass container with an airtight lid.

Serve with berries, soy yogurt natural milk.

SPINACH TOFU BENEDICT WITH VEGAN HOLLANDAISE

This benign spinach tofu will satisfy your desire for a cozy coffee without eating eggs. Delicious, coffee, or a simple dinner recipe, this Spinach Tofu with Vegan Hollandaise Sauce is packed with plant-based nutrition!

BENEDICT WITH VEGAN HOLLANDAISE

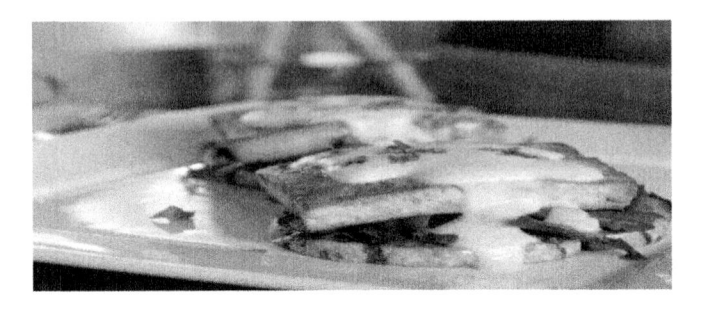

To replace the English muffin, use this vegan Benedictine recipe Pumpkin. This pumpkin rich in carotenoids has anti-carcinogenic, anti-inflammatory, and antioxidant compounds that make it possible to prevent cancer.

Of course, you can use a traditional English muffin instead of a pumpkin for this vegan tofu if you want.

Dark, rich green vegetables such as Swiss chard, cabbage, kale, or spinach are also used to layer this nutrient-poor breakfast. Green vegetables are full of minerals, vitamins, pigments, and phytonutrients including potassium, manganese, zinc, magnesium, iron, and calcium.

VEGAN RECIPE ONLY

In a small saucepan, add 1/4 cup non-skimmed milk and pour the flour and turmeric over medium heat. Add the remaining 3/4 cup milk. Add lemon juice, salt, and pepper to taste. The sauce starts to thicken if you contradict it when boiling.

Take the vegan hollandaise recipe from the heat and add the Dijon mustard to the nearest dish.

VEGETAL ADVANTAGE

Put about 3 slices of pumpkin on your plate and garnish with 1/2 cup spinach. Afterward, a piece of tofu and dried with simple vegan hollandaise sauces are dried. I love serving mine with a nice cut of whole-grain toast!

Ingredients

1 container of 16 oz. of tofu, served in 8 1/2 plates

1/4 cup Tamari (like soy sauce)

1 Tbl Worcestershire Vegan

2 c. 1 teaspoon of syrup

1/2 teaspoon optional liquid steam

10 oz fresh or frozen spinach

Wash 1 squash, cut in half and remove the seeds (no need to peel)

Add salt and pepper to taste

Hollandaise Zoos

1 cup non-dairy milk

1 1 / 2-2 Tbl unbleached flour (for gluten-free, use rice flour)

1/8 teaspoon turmeric

4 tablespoons lemon juice

1 tablespoon of food allergen

1/2 tablespoon Dijon mustard

1/4 teaspoon sea salt

Serve with spinach and tofu

Instructions

For the tofu:

Mix the tamari, Worcestershire vegan sauces, the maple syrup, and the liquid stream in the tofu container and bring the tofu slices into the marinade for a few minutes.

Once the tofu has marinated for a few minutes to 30 minutes, place it in a non-stick pan over medium heat and cook until brown on one side, about 5 minutes. Flip and brown on the other side. Lay on the side.

Squash

Wash and cut in half and remove the seeds (keep the seeds to run if you want).

Turn the pumpkin over and cut it into 1/2 inch slices. Place on a baking sheet, cut with parchment paper. Sprinkle with salt and pepper.

Bake for 15 minutes, flip and bake for another 15 minutes or until done. Sit when done.

Dutch:

In a small saucepan, add about 1/4 cup non-dairy milk and squeeze the turmeric and flour.

Over medium heat, whisk the mixture while adding the rest of the non-skimmed milk.

Add salt, lemon juice, and pepper to taste. Continue until the sauce thickens. If it is not thick enough, you should add a little more flour with non-skimmed milk in a separate container and whisk, or shake if you have a blanket, and add it to the sauce.

Remove from heat and add Dijon mustard to the food bowl. Whisk to combine. If the sauce is too thick, add a little or more water or non-skimmed milk.

To collect: Two servings of tofu each. Place a few slices of delicate pumpkin (about 3) in two separate areas of the plate. Garnish with about 1/2 cup spinach each. Garnish the spinach with a slice of tofu and then the hollandaise sauce. Sprinkle with parsley for garnish.

Serve with strong whole-grain toast.

OVERNIGHT CHIA OATS

Mornings can be stressful and these evenings are a great solution in the early morning! They help you stay on track and if you have several servings at a time, your week is set. Not only that, but the addition of chia seeds contains heart-healthy omega-3 fatty acids.

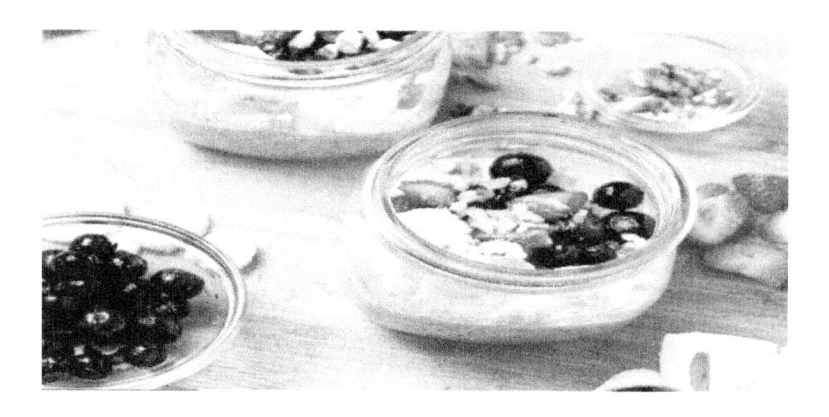

Then just add the chia seeds, oatmeal, non-skim milk, cinnamon, vanilla, and a pinch of salt. Clean well, cover, and cool overnight. In the morning, mix fruit and some nuts and tree, your coffee are ready.

A serving of oatmeal is only cooked 1/2 cup and that may not seem like enough. These pint-sized warriors are perfect if you need to add something.

Chia Oats overnight in Mason Jars with fresh berries

Ingredients

1/4 cup old peeled oats

1/2 cup unsweetened Milk OR Three trees house almond milk

1/4 teaspoon. 1 teaspoon Ceylon Cinnamon

1/4 teaspoon vanilla extract

2 tablespoons white chia seeds

1/2 tablespoon maple syrup

1/4 cup fresh or frozen blueberries

1/4 cup fresh or frozen strawberries

5 oz nuts

Instructions

For each jar contain (1/4 cup oats, 1/2 cup milk, 1/4 teaspoon cinnamon and vanilla, 2 tablespoons chia acids, 1/2 tablespoon maple syrup)

CHAPTER FOUR

SOUP

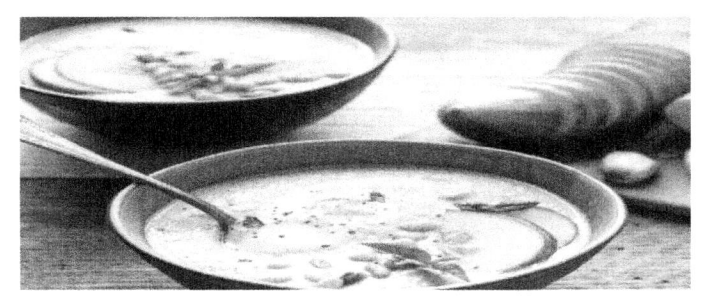

Ingredients

3 English cucumbers (2 lbs in total), peeled

1 1/2 yellow peppers, cut into 1/4 inch cubes

1 1/2 fresh jalapeño pepper, sautéed and chopped

1 large garlic clove, chopped

3 tablespoons fresh lemon juice

3/4 cup chopped fresh coriander

3/4 cup sour cream

1 teaspoon salt

1/4 teaspoon black pepper

Ingredients

1 cup (150 g) raw cashews, cooked overnight

2 cucumbers (about 650 g)

1/4 cup (60 ml) whole coconut milk

2 tablespoons (30g) Basil Pesto

2 tablespoons (30 ml) lemon juice

1 C. 1 tablespoon (17g) white miso

1 tablespoon (15 ml) maple syrup

2 garlic cloves

1/4 teaspoon salt

1/8 teaspoon mixed black pepper

4-5 mint leaves

Garnish: cucumber slices, roasted pine nuts, basil leaves

Instructions

Wash the cucumbers. Cut them in half and screw the seeds with a teaspoon. Chop the cucumbers and place them in a high-speed mixer.

Drain the cashews and add them to the mixer with all the other ingredients: coconut milk, pesto, lemon juice, miso, maple syrup, garlic, salt, chopped pepper, and mint leaves.

Blend on high speed for 1 to 2 minutes or until very smooth. Taste and adjust the seasons if necessary. For a good kick, add a pinch of red pepper flakes.

Transfer to a large bowl or saucepan, cover, and refrigerate for at least 2 hours before serving.

Serve freshly garnished with cucumber slices, grilled pine nuts, and fresh basil. The soup stays in the fridge for up to 3 days.

MUSHROOM SOUP

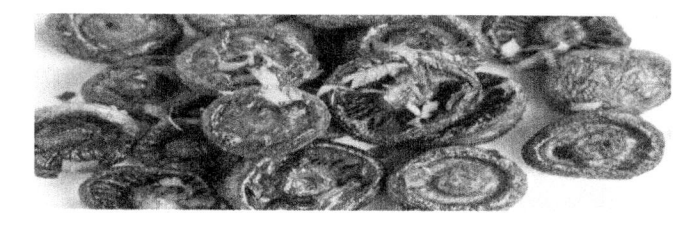

Ingredients

2 tablespoons butter

1/2 pound sliced fresh mushrooms

1/4 cup chopped onion

6 tablespoons whole purpose flour

1/2 teaspoon salt

1/8 teaspoon pepper

2 cans of Chicken broth (1 / 2 ounces each)

1 cup half and half cream

Instructions

In a large saucepan, heat the butter over medium-high heat; sauté mushrooms and onion until tender.

Stir the flour, salt, pepper with 1 can of broth until smooth; add the mushroom mixture. Stir in the rest of the broth. Cook and stir until thickened, for 2 minutes. Lower the temperature; adds the cream. Simmer, uncovered, until the mixture is mixed, about 15 minutes, stirring occasionally.

Many people do not know the difference between chicken broth and chicken broth. Chicken broth is made of bone, while the chicken broth is made of meat.

Mushrooms are rich in vitamin B, which makes them a great advocate for heart health.

VEGAN CLAM CHOWDER

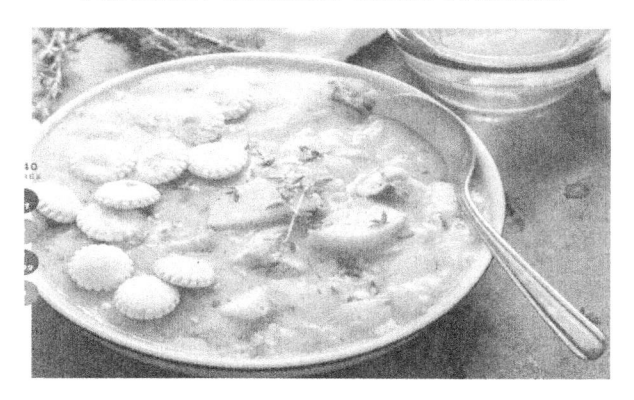

Ingredients

2 tablespoons vegan butter, divided

4 ounces shiitake mushroom caps, coarsely chopped

1 medium onion, chopped

2 medium celery sticks, chopped

3 garlic cloves, chopped

3 tablespoons whole purpose flour

3/4 cup dry white wine

2 cups low sodium vegetable broth

1 1/4 cup light coconut milk

1 pound with golden potatoes, ripe and cut into 1 inch pieces

1 tablespoon Dulse blacken

1 teaspoon dried thyme leaves

2 bay leaves

2 tablespoons white miso paste

1 teaspoon white wine vinegar

Season with salt and pepper

Serving (optional)

Oysters or salt crackers

Coconut Bacon

Instructions

Make a large saucepan over medium heat and add 1 tablespoon of vegan butter.

When the butter has melted, add the shiitake mushrooms in a relatively even layer. Stir a few times to melt the mushrooms, cook them for about 4 minutes, until golden on the ground.

Allow the pineapple to simmer and cook for about 4 more minutes, then brown on opposite sides.

Remove the mushrooms from the pan and transfer them to a plate.

Melt the remaining tablespoons of butter in the pan, add the celery and onion.

Cook celery and onion for about 5 minutes, stirring occasionally, until soft and translucent.

Add the garlic and flour to the pot and toss the vegetables with the flour. Cook for about 2 minutes, turning regularly.

Fry the wine and bring to the boil. Cook for about 3 minutes.

Stir in broth, coconut milk, potatoes, dill, thyme, and bay leaves. Return the mushrooms to the pot. Raise the heat, bring the liquid to a boil, then reduce the heat to a boil.

Simmer the mixture until the potatoes are softened, about 12 to 15 minutes.

Pour a small amount of the liquid from the jar into a small bowl and add the miso paste.

Whisk until mixed, then stir the mixture into the pot.

Remove the bay leaves from the soup.

Stir in the vinegar, test the taste and season with S&P to taste. You can also optionally mix a small amount (1 cup) with a blender, or stick a dew blender in the jar for a second or two.

Put in bowls and garnish with sides of your choice.

CHAPTER FIVE

TOMATOES BEAN SOUP

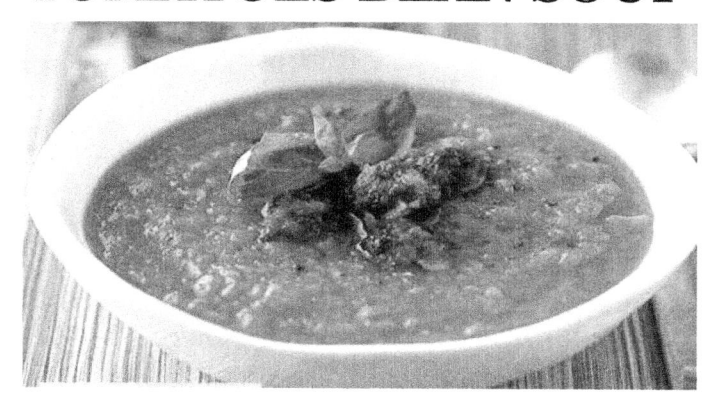

Spicy Tomato and Bean Soup is the perfect lunch break or for work lunch. It heats up very well and fills up due to the beans.

We recommend using baked beans to use your spicy beans in tomato soup (who doesn't have a can in the cupboard?), Then add crushed chili flakes on top for a bit of foot chic. Of course, these can be removed if you also have small mouths that eat. To enjoy fresh and crispy bread, preferably warm from the oven.

Ingredients

415g baked beans

2 tablespoons vegetables

1 onion, coarsely chopped

125 g (4 oz.) Chopped celery

1 clove garlic, crushed

2 tablespoons dried mixed herbs

1 tablespoon dried crushed pepper

400 g (chopped) tomatoes

600 ml (1 pt) vegetable broth

To serve:

4 tablespoons cream

Toast

Instruction

Heat the oil in a deep-frying saucepan. Add the onion, celery, garlic, herb mixture, and chili and cook for about 5 minutes on medium heat. Add the tomatoes, baked beans, and broth to the pan. Cover and simmer for 25 minutes.

Serve the soup in hot bowls, seasoned with a whisk of sour cream, and accompanied by slices of bread.

SAUTEED KALE SALAD

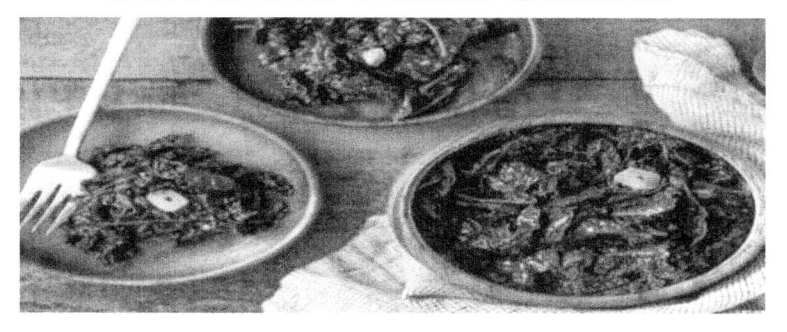

This kale, which is fried with garlic and olive oil, is lightly shaken by the red pepper flakes. It's a fantastic side dish and turns into a meal when mixed with pasta Slideshow: Recipes for greens

Ingredients

3 tablespoons extra virgin olive oil 3 garlic cloves, thinly sliced 1/4 teaspoon red pepper flakes 2 volumes cold, cleaned and dried, ribs and stalks removed, leaves thinly sliced kosher salt Freshly ground black pepper

Step 1

In pot oven, heat the oil over average hot. Add the garlic and chili flakes and sauté for two minutes until the garlic just starts to brown.

Step 2

Add the kale to batches and drain with oil. Once all the kale has been added to the pan, cover, and sauté for 5 minutes.

Stage 3

Remove the cover, cover with salt and pepper, and cook for another three minutes or until the moisture has evaporated. Serve immediately.

WARM BALSAMIC KALE SALAD

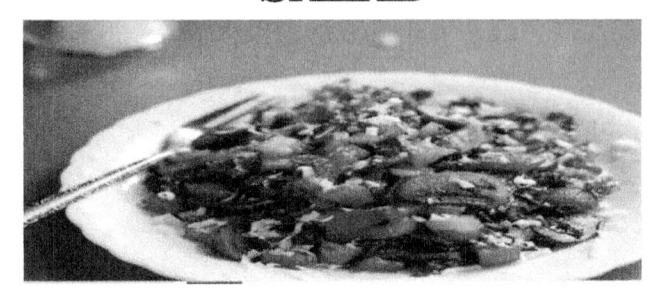

This warm balsamic kale salad has tons of flavor and contains sour soups and peppers, and cheese.

Ingredients

2 tablespoons butter

1/4 cup tipped onion

1 red pepper, diced

1 yellow pepper, diced

8-ounce baby Portobello mushrooms, sliced

4 Cups Kale

1 teaspoon garlic, chopped

1 tablespoon balsamic vinegar

1/4 cup cheese

Salt and pepper to taste

Instructions

In a large skillet over medium heat, melt a tablespoon of butter. Add the onions and peppers; sauté for a few minutes until softened. Add mushrooms to a tablespoon of butter; sauté for a few minutes until golden brown.

Add the kale, garlic, and balsamic vinegar. Sauté until the cabbage is dark green but not yet faded. Remove from the heat and serve topped with Parmesan cheese. To taste well sandwich with salt and pepper.

STRAWBERRY DANDELION SALAD

Lion varieties of green are good enough for you rich in calcium, iron, and antioxidants.

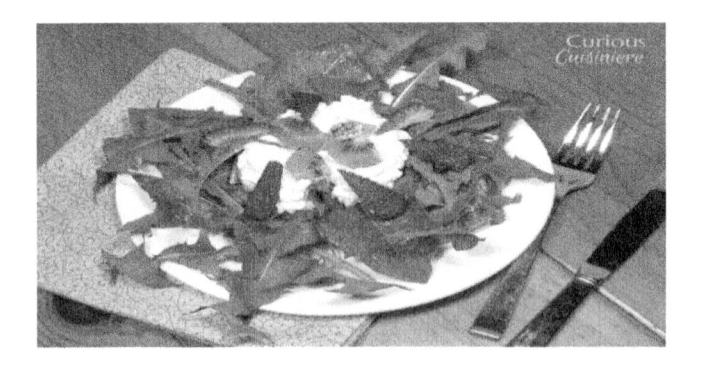

Have you ever had a lion salad? Lion leaves are a unique spicy addition to this spring salad!

Ingredients

2 large handfuls of dandelion leaves

4 large romaine lettuce leaves

2-3 large strawberries

1 Kiwi

1/3 teaspoon cottage cheese

Your Favorite Fruity Vinaigrette

Instructions

Wash the vegetables thoroughly and cut them into small pieces.

Take off your boots and slice the strawberries.

Remove the nut, grate it and press the juice.

Put a bed of green vegetables on your wallet. Garnish with cottage cheese and fruit.

Add the dressing. Mix and enjoy

RAINBOW SALAD

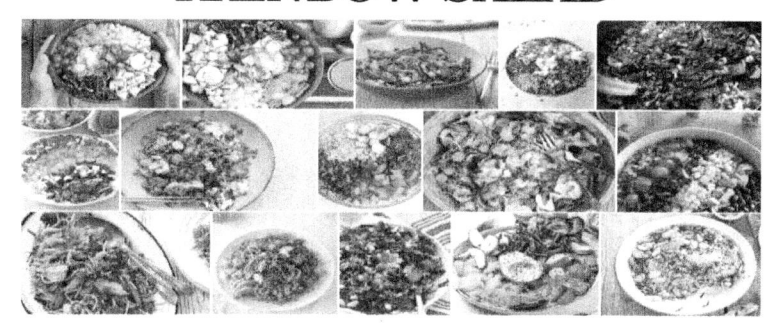

REASON FOR RAINBOW SALAD

By choosing foods of all colors of the rainbow, you maximize the number of different micronutrients you eat. It's very important. Sometimes we can stick to the same vegetables over and over again, but it's important to diversify what we eat to make sure we're getting all the nutrients we need.

Brightly colored fruits and vegetables are rich in antioxidants that protect us from free radicals and help disease among others.

CHOOSE A DARK GREEN BASE

For the base of your salad, you want to choose a dark, pale green like spinach, kale, Swiss chard, kale, or a combination of one or other greens. You can also choose mixed salad greens, but I prefer warmer greens than kale because they last better after dressing.

Cold (red, green or black)

Spinach

Swiss sharp

green mesclun

Mustard green

curled salad

green cabbage

If you eat your salad right away with no leftovers, then the greens work great, if you plan to eat it the next day, then I would go with something like kale chard.

I used a mixture of spinach and kale for my base.

NUTRITION BENEFITS OF DARK GROUND AND LOSE

Green leafy vegetables are rich in nutrients and one of the healthiest foods you can eat. They are a vital source of antioxidants, fiber, and phytonutrients, help prevent the disease and promote good digestion, brain, and heart health. Green Vegetable Vegetables are rich in vitamins A, C, K, and folic acid and minerals of calcium, iron, potassium, and magnesium. They are also very low in calories, so you can go ahead and refuel to create foods that are low in calories but rich in nutrients.

Healthy daily rainbow salad with ginger and sweet miso vinaigrette

RED PURPLE VEGETABLES

Diced tomatoes sun-dried would be nice too

tipped red pepper or grilled red pepper

thinly sliced radish

grilled, steamed or roasted raw beets red, striped or golden) finely chopped Radicchio

finely chopped red cabbage

Roasted Oven (Purple Yam)

tipped red onion, thinly sliced, marinated or roasted

I used raw roasted beets and thinly sliced red cabbage.

NUTRITIONAL NAMES OF RED VEGETABLES AND PURPLE

The phytonutrients that color red and purple vegetables come with powerful health benefits. Deeper, richer colors mean vegetables are rich in phytonutrients such as antioxidants, vitamins, and minerals, and these nutrients have been shown to prevent cancer, fight chronic diseases, and strengthen the immune system.

Red vegetables get their color from lycopene and anthocyanin. Lycopene is an important antioxidant that has been shown to reduce heart disease, promote eye health, and fight infections. Anthocyanins, which are also found in violet vegetables such as purple cabbage, help protect the liver, reduce blood pressure, and have anti-inflammatory properties.

ORANGE AND VEGETABLES

grated carrot

tipped orange pepper

Roasted butternut squash, baked or steamed

Roasted kabocha pumpkin, baked or steamed

fried cubed sweet potatoes, baked or steamed

roasted, baked or steamed acorn

diced yellow Pepper

yellow Summer Squash

grated golden beets

BENEFITS OF ORANGE AND YELLOW VEGETABLES

All of these vegetables have their unique nutritional profile, but as a group, these brightly colored vegetables contain zeaxanthin, flavonoids, lycopene, potassium, vitamin C, and beta-carotene. Nutrients help our body in various ways, from reducing the risk of macular degeneration to protecting the bones.

GREEN VEGETABLES

Raw, steamed or fried broccoli

Cube of green pepper

tipped cucumbers

spicy zucchini

Chickpeas

all kinds of sprouts (broccoli, alfalfa, etc.)

finely chopped or grated green cabbage

I used steamed broccoli.

NUTRITIONAL BENEFITS OF GREEN VEGETABLES

Just like leafy vegetables, green vegetables are usually rich in vitamin C and contain vitamins A, K, calcium, potassium, and iron, and of course are a great source of fiber. Cabbages, sprouts, and broccoli are particularly rich in nutrients, so try to include as much as possible, especially broccoli. The many nutrients found in green vegetables are important for a healthy immune system, cardiovascular health, and disease prevention.

In addition to all these general benefits, each fruit and vegetable has its specific nutritional profile, which is why the daily consumption of a wide range of plants is so important for your overall health. The list of vegetables I have provided is not exhaustive but contains the most common and most available. There are so many others you can add to salads, think fennel, endive, fresh herbs, kohlrabi, turnips, artichokes, and watercress, to name a few - one!

WHAT ABOUT FRUIT?

I don't always eat fruits for my daily salads, but they do add sweetness to their nutritional benefits. If you want to add colorful fruits, I would recommend:

Fresh berries like blueberry, strawberry or blackberry

chopped apples or pears

chopped orange or grapefruit

Grenade

sliced papaya or mango

cut peach or nectarine

chopped kiwi

chopped watermelon

I like fresh berries and sliced stone fruits like nectarine when they are in season, otherwise, I would say pomegranates, apples, and pears are my favorites. I did not add any fruit to this salad, but chopped apples or plums would be great.

CHAPTER SIX

AVOCADO SAUCE

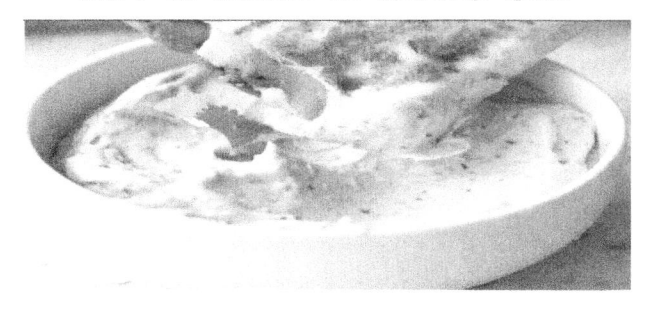

Health Benefits of Avocado

An avocado sauce is a much healthier option than a dip loaded with mayo! Avocado is full of vitamins, minerals, fiber, and healthy fats! One of the few natural products that contain a significant amount of monounsaturated fatty acids. These are good fats, which lower cholesterol and support heart health.

With nearly 20 vitamins and minerals, their potential health benefits include improved digestion, good for the heart, low cholesterol, low risk of depression, and protection against cancer. Avocado is also good for weight loss because it is rich in fiber. Fats that will keep you going longer. You are much better offloading avocado salad than cheese, or roasting avocado on your morning toast instead of peanut butter! But since they contain 77% fat, they should be consumed in moderation.

Ingredients

1 large ripe avocado

1/3 cup sour cream or yogurt

1/2 small garlic cloves

1/2 lemon juice

1-2 tablespoons olive oil

1/2 cup (packed) Cilantro Coriander, rough chopped

Season with salt and pepper

Instructions

Mix all the ingredients in a food processor, mixing until very smooth. Use water to adjust the consistency as needed.

Adjust the lemon or lime if necessary. Should have a bit of flavor when paired with rich and fatty foods like Mexican food.

Keep 4 days in an airtight container - and stay green!

CHEESE SAUCE

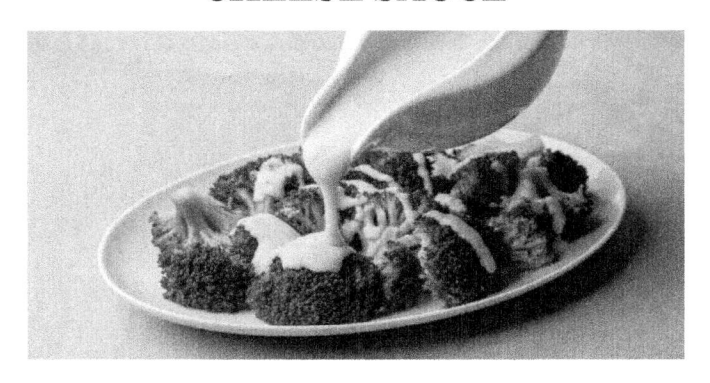

Ingredients

3 tablespoons butter

3 tablespoons whole purpose flour

1/2 teaspoon salt

1/4 teaspoon dry mustard

1/8 teaspoon grated black pepper (or white pepper)

1 1/2 cups milk (or light cream)

1 cup grated cheddar cheese (soft or spicy)

Preparation

 Ingredients for a simple cheddar cheese sauce

Melt the butter in a saucepan over medium-low heat; extinguish the fire. Stir in the flour, salt, dry mustard, and pepper.

Add and mix in the melted butter, flour, salt, dry mustard, and pepper

Put the pan on the heat and cook for 1 minute, stirring.

Stir while heating the butter-flour mixture

Slowly add milk or light cream, stirring until combined.

Milk is added and stirred with a wooden spoon

Continue to cook, stirring constantly, until thickened and creamy. Simmer for 5 minutes as you lower the heat.

Stir until a mixture becomes thick and smooth

Add cheese and cook, stirring constantly, until cheese is melted and the sauce is smooth and well combined.

Add grilled cheddar cheese and stir until melted and smooth

Serve with pasta or vegetables and enjoy.

GARLIC SAUCE

What is Garlic Sauce Made of?

Garlic: The most important part of the recipe is garlic. Find the freshest garlic cloves you can find. Test their firmness to make sure they have the best consistency and taste. You will need a cup of peeled garlic. You can freeze the remaining garlic.

Oil: You can use canola oil, vegetable oil, saffron oil, avocado oil, grape juice oil, or any neutral oil you want. I do not recommend using olive oil as it will change the color of the garlic sauce and give it a stronger taste than the neutral oil. You want the aroma of garlic to last longer than the aroma of the oil. You will need 3 to 4 cups of oil.

Lemon juice: Lemon plays a supporting role in Lebanese garlic sauce and helps to bind and emulsify so that the oil does not dominate the garlic. I use 1/2 cup but you can take off to your liking. Lemon juice acts as a binder, so remember.

Salt: Salt helps to veneer the garlic by adding traction to the natural moisture of the garlic at the beginning of the treatment. Plus, it helps to taste the sauce.

HOW TO MAKE GARLIC SAUCE HOMEMADE

Remove the green sprout from the inside of the garlic. This step is not necessary, but make sure you remove the oldest part of the garlic to leave with the coolest and whitest part of the garlic. The result is a less bitter sauce, so it's worth it if you have the time.

Soak the garlic in ice water for a few minutes for a less potent taste. Some readers have mentioned that the taste of garlic is really strong. One way to reduce this potency is to immerse the garlic in ice water. Be sure to dry them afterward when doing so.

Be sure to alternate the lemon juice with the oil. I have seen the garlic sauce a few times as I tried to leave the lemon juice until the end, but the oil becomes too hard to support the garlic like that. Lemon juice helps to keep the consistency light, so I suggest it alternately as soon as the mixture is initially emulsified.

Do not use a mixer. It is really difficult to emulsify the mixture in a standard mixer or a defrost blender. A mixer also does not allow the oil to be sipped slowly while the engine is running over a large area. I do not recommend a mixer.

Ingredients

1 cup peeled garlic cloves

2 teaspoons kosher salt

3 cups neutral oil like canola or saffron

½ Cup of Lemon Juice

Instructions

Cut the garlic cloves in half lengthwise and remove the green sprouts.

Transfer the sliced garlic slices to a food processor and add the kosher salt to the garlic slices. Mix for a minute until the garlic is finely chopped. Then make sure to screw the sides of the food processor.

Run with the food processor, slowly fry one to two tablespoons of oil, then stop and unscrew the bowl. Continue adding a tablespoon or two until the garlic starts to look creamy.

When the onion seems to be emulsified by a few tablespoons of oil, increase the speed of pouring the oil and alternate with the 1/2 cup of lemon juice until all the oil is integrated into the lemon juice. It takes about 15 minutes. Put the sauce in a glass container and cover it with a paper towel in the fridge overnight.

The next day, replace the paper towel with a tight-fitting lid and store it in the fridge for up to 3 months.

What to eat with garlic sauce

The possibilities for serving tum are endless. We especially like it with grilled meat and chicken. But it works very well with grilled fish, and sandwiches, and pasta. It also works as a dip with pita bread and crackers. Or you can use it as a base for a garlic vinaigrette. Here are some great recipes that work with garlic sauce.

Chicken Rolls

Chicken Shawarma Zalot

Roasted Cauliflower Pitas

Shawarma Pizza Pita

HOW TO MAKE HOMEMADE BARBEQUE SAUCE

Ingredients

1 tablespoon olive oil

2 garlic cloves, chopped

1 8 Oz Tomato Sauce

1/2 teaspoon granulated onion

2 tablespoons tomato paste

2 tablespoons molasses

1 1/2 tablespoons raw honey

1 tablespoon apple cider vinegar

1/4 teaspoon sea salt

1/4 teaspoon. 1 teaspoon black pepper

Instructions

Heat olive oil over medium-high heat in a saucepan, then add the chopped garlic.

Cook for a minute until the garlic is perfumed, then add tomato sauce, tomato paste, molasses, raw honey, apple cider vinegar, granulated onion, sea salt, and black pepper, and stir to combine.

CHAPTER SEVEN

WALNUT MILK

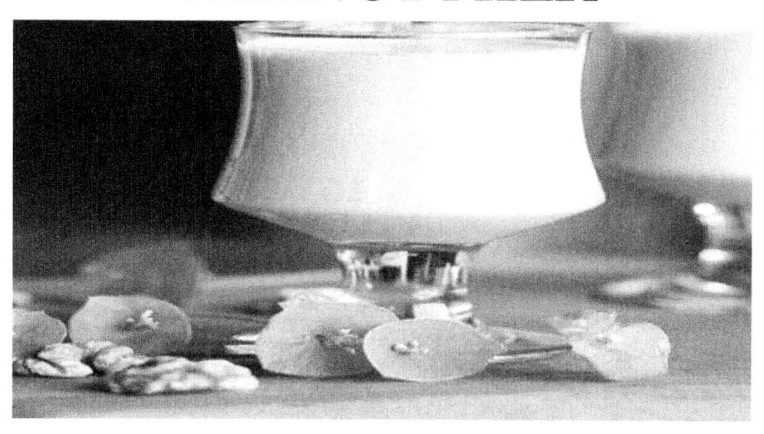

Nut and brain health

I was surprised to find that nuts contain melatonin. Melatonin is a hormone secreted by the pineal gland that regulates your sleep-wake cycle, promoting a healthy sleep (which in turn supports healthy, alarming brain function).

Nuts are rich in vitamin E. This antioxidant quality of super vitamin E means better brain health. Vitamin E is believed to help with oxidative stress and damage to the brain. Low levels of vitamin E have even been linked to Alzheimer's disease. Omega-3s (which are rich in nuts) are also known to support overall brain health and improve cognitive function.

Nuts and circulatory system support

Walnuts have the amino acid L-Arginine, which is known to support the vascular system. The vascular system is better known as the circulatory system, which consists of the vessels responsible for transporting blood and lymph fluid in the body. The arteries and veins in this system carry oxygen and nutrients throughout the body, causing unwanted tissue.

Nuts for a healthy heart and cholesterol levels

Nuts are one of the best sources of plant-derived omega-3 essential fatty acids, in the form of alpha-linolenic acid (ALA). Not only does omega-3 support a healthy brain, but ALA is also important for helping the body maintain a healthy cholesterol level. ALA is great for heart health because it can help lower blood pressure, prevent heart attacks, and reverse atherosclerosis (hardening of the arteries).

Research shows that linoleic acid is believed to reduce the risk of heart disease by maintaining a normal heart rate and a normal heart rate. It could also reduce blood clots.

Make vegetable milk with nuts

Emergency milk is one of the healthiest plant-based milk out there. It's ridiculously simple and offers a great way to get a very useful dose of nuts into your system. Making milk with seed means that they have been scaled down and are likely easier to assimilate into your system (although I recommend using them for other plant-based recipes as well such as superfood brownies).

Raw and other delicacies!

You can soak your nuts overnight (or for a few hours to soften them). You can also go ahead and not suck at all if you forgot or want to save nuts. So there is no real excuse.

You do not need a nice high-power mixer - a cheap, inexpensive mixer will do just fine.

A bag of nuts or something similar?

A bag of nuts is recommended for straining muslin or gauze, which only takes a minute. Bags of milk are not expensive. Cloth, cotton hemp bags are harder to clean, so I recommend a nylon-type mother bag that will last a very long time and is very easy to rinse after use See the recipe below for some nut bag suggestions.

Ingredients

100g (1 cup nuts)

750 ml (about 3 cups) of water

A hint of vanilla (optional)

1 tablespoon coconut sugar (optional but tasty)

Instructions

Leave the nuts overnight to soak them for a few hours. You can also mix it without drinking the nuts are a little harder, that's all if you forgot or do not have time to push.

Drain and then rinse with water.

Put into a mixing bowl, add about 750 ml (about 3 cups) of pure water, and mix for about a minute. It works in a cheap blender or a powerful blender.

Strain the mixed milk into a bag of the nuts press.

Pour into a glass bottle, cup or jar. Open the lid and let it cool in the fridge.

PAPAYA SEED DRESSING

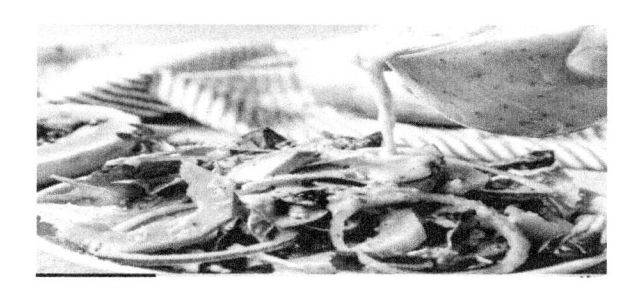

HOW TO PREPARE PAPAYA

If you, like me, do not have much experience with papaya, prepare it as you would a cantaloupe.

Cut the whole thing in half lengthwise, then clean the seeds with a spoon. Normally I just throw them in the trash, like with cantaloupe seeds, but now that I know better, I remove the saws for this papaya seed dressing and reserve.

Then you just need to use a sharp knife to remove the flesh from the fruit of the thick skin and cut or slice to serve.

PAPAYA SED DRESSING
INGREDIENTS

Rice vinegar

Canola Oil

Sweet onion

Honey

Salt

Dry mustard

Fresh papaya seeds

HOW TO MAKE A PAPAYA SEED DRESSING

Combine vinegar, oil, chopped onion, sugar, salt, and mustard until smooth in a blender, then papaya seeds and mix until similar to peppercorns. Coarse soil.

In a large bowl or on individual serving plates, toss the greens of your choice with chopped red onions, avocado, and papaya. Drizzle with a little vinaigrette and toss to coat.

Papaya Seed Dressing with Coconut Cashews and Spinach Salad

This classic, tangy Hawaiian vinaigrette adds a peppery touch to ground papaya seeds. Most papaya seed dressings are high in sugar. Here the dried mango replaces most of the sugar. This elegant main course salad is perfect to pair. I'm a big fan of Rancho Gordo Stardust Dip Powder. It is perfect for sweet or savory dishes.

Spinach Salad with Papaya Seed and Coconut Cashew Vinaigrette

Put the champagne vinegar, dried mango, and scallions in a blender and reduce to a smooth puree. Add the agave nectar, Dijon mustard, ginger, salt and pepper, and mix. Add the papaya seeds and avocado oil and mix again.

Prepare the Coconut Cashews Place the cashews in a medium bowl. Add the melted coconut oil, agave, and coconut sugar and mix well. Add the coconut flakes to the Stardust pepper powder and stir until combined. On a large skillet over medium heat, sauté the mixture until golden brown. Place on a sheet of baking paper, distribute evenly and allow to cool to room temperature.

Peel and cut the red end. Dip them into a bowl of ice water. Let it sit for at least ten minutes, stirring once or twice, reducing and drying on a kitchen towel.

Prepare the salad - In a large flat bowl, place on the spinach. Add 2 tablespoons of the dressing and mix. Garnish with chopped papaya and chopped red onion. Garnish with the toasted coconut cashews. Serve with a fresh baguette and additional dressing.

CUCUMBER DILL SAUCE

Ingredients

1 medium cucumber, peeled, sliced, and cut into 1/4-inch pieces

1/2 teaspoon salt

3/4 cup sour cream

2 tablespoons whole milk

2 tablespoons chopped fresh dill

Preparation

Combine the cucumbers with 1/2 teaspoon of salt in a medium bowl. Let stand 30 minutes. Transfer to a colander and rinse well. Pat the cucumbers dry with paper towels.

Combine cucumber, sour cream, milk, and dill in a small bowl. Season with salt and pepper. Cover and refrigerate for 2 hours. Can be prepared one day in advance. Store in the refrigerator.

Ingredients

1/4 cup low fat sour cream

2 tablespoons mayonnaise

Juice and zest of 1/2 lemon

3 tablespoons peeled, sown and finely dried cucumbers

1/2 small green onion, sliced

1 tablespoon chopped fresh dill

1 clove garlic, chopped

Add salt and freshly ground pepper to taste

Get ingredients powered by chicory

Instructions

Combine mayonnaise, sour cream, cucumber, fresh dill, green onion, lemon juice, chopped garlic, sea salt, and freshly ground pepper to taste in a bowl. Mix until well blended. Refrigerate until ready to use. Enjoy.

CHAPTER EIGHT

BREAD AND SNACKS

SEED CRACKERS

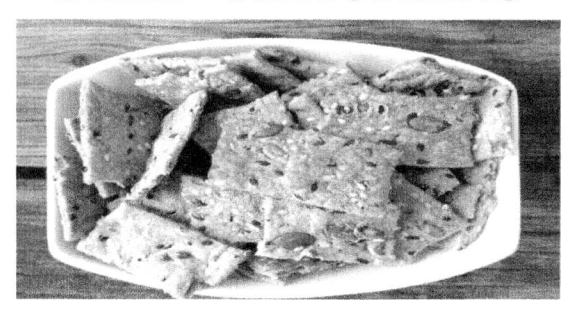

Ingredients

250 grams of strong white bread flour or any purpose flour

25 grams of pumpkin seeds

25 Grams of Flax Somen

25 grams of sunflower names

15 grams of sesame seeds

5 grams of mussels

50 grams of olive oil

5 grams of fine acid salt

100 grams of water

Instructions

Preheat the oven to 335F; knit two baking sheets with parchment paper and set them up

Know the ingredients in the mixing bowl; combine for 15 seconds with speed 3

Knead for 1 minute and 30 seconds; switch to a lightly maintained work surface

Cut the dough in half; roll out each portion very thinly (1-2 mm)

Cut into squares or rectangles or use a cooking cutter circle; Place on the prepared baking sheet

Bake for 20-25 minutes; cool and store in an airtight container

TORTILLAS HOMEMADE

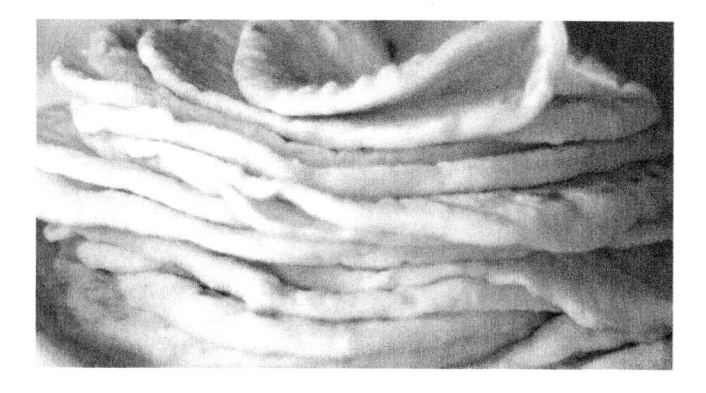

Ingredients

3 cups whole purpose

1 teaspoon salt

1 teaspoon baking powder

⅓ Cup extra virgin olive oil, vegetable oil or other fairly neutral-flavored oil

1 cup of happy water

Instructions

Put together flour, baking powder, and salt in the bowl of a mixer. Using the dough hook, mix the dry ingredients until well combined.

Add oil and water to the mixer on medium speed. After about 1 minute, or when the mixture comes together and begins to form a ball, reduce the mixing speed to low. Continue to mix for a minute or until the dough is smooth.

Transfer the dough to a lightly flattened work surface. Divide into 16 equal portions. Make each piece to layer with flour. Form each piece into a ball and flatten it with the palm of your hand. Cover the flat balls of the dough with a clean kitchen towel and leave for at least 15 minutes (or up to 2 hours) before continuing.

After serving, heat a large skillet over medium heat. Roll each piece of dough into a diameter around 6-7 inches in diameter, keeping the work surface and roll lightly cared for. Do not stack the raw tortillas together, otherwise, they will stick together.

When the pot is hot, place a circle of dough in the pan and cook for about 1 minute or until the bottom surface has some light brown spots and the uncooked surface bubbles. If the spread is too fast, reduce the heat a bit. If it takes more than a minute to see some bright golden brown spots on the end of the tortillas, the heat increases a bit. Flip to the other side and cook for 15 to 20 seconds. The tortillas should be nice and soft but have some small brown spots on the surface.

Remove from the pan with tongs and stack in a covered container or zippered bag to keep the tortillas soft.

Serve warm or allow to cool to use later. When ready to use, place a slightly damp paper towel in the bottom of a microwave-safe container (with a lid) that holds the stacked tortillas. Microwave uncovered for 15 to 30 seconds (starting at 15) or until heated through, then cover to retain heat while serving.

Store in an airtight container or zippered bag with room temperature for 24 hours or in the refrigerator for up to 1 week. To freeze, separate the tortillas with parchment or white paper and place them in a zippered bag before placing them in the freezer.

TORTILLAS CHIPS

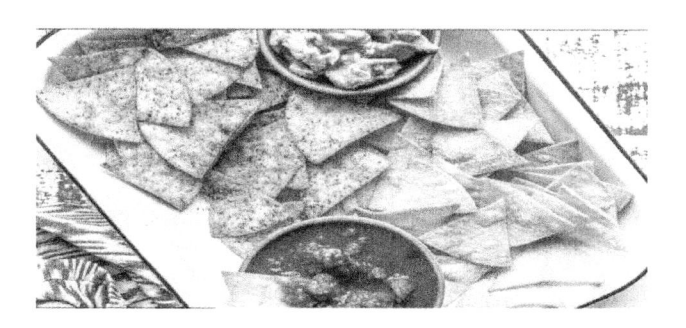

12 ounces) Package of Tortillas

1 tablespoon vegetable oil

3 tablespoons lemon juice

1 teaspoon of ground cumin

1 teaspoon chili powder

1 teaspoon salt

Add all ingredients to the shopping (12 ounces) Package of Tortillas

1 tablespoon vegetable oil

3 tablespoons lemon juice

1 teaspoon of ground cumin

1 teaspoon chili powder

1 teaspoon salt

Add all ingredients to the shopping list

Step 1

Preheat the oven to 175 ° C.

Step 2

Cut each tortilla into 8 chip-sized wedges and arrange the wedges in a single layer on a baking sheet.

Stage 3

In a sprayer, combine the oil and the lime juice. Mix well and sprinkle each tortilla wedge until slightly moist.

Step 4

Combine cumin, chili powder, and salt in a small bowl and sprinkle over the chips.

Step 5

Bake for about 7 minutes. Remove the pan and cook for another 8 minutes or until the chips are crispy, but not too thick. Serve with salsas, garnish, or guacamole.

CHAPTER NINE

FOOD TO AVOID

It is easy to confuse which foods are healthy and which are not. In general, you want to avoid certain foods if you want to lose weight and prevent chronic diseases.

20 Unhealthy foods

Well, most people can eat them in moderation on special occasions without permanent damage to their health.

Sugary drinks

Adding sugar to ingredients is bad in the modern diet. However, some sources of sugar are worse than others, and sugary drinks are especially harmful. When you drink liquid calories, your brain does not seem to record them as food. Thus, you can drastically increase your total calorie intake When consumed in large quantities, sugar can increase insulin resistance and is closely linked to non-alcoholic fatty liver. It is also associated with several serious conditions, such as type 2 diabetes and heart disease

Some people believe that sugary drinks are the most important fact in the modern diet and consuming them in large quantities can cause fat gain and obesity

Alternatives

Instead, drink water, carbonated water, coffee, or tea. Adding a slice of lemon to water or carbonated water can add a flavor.

2. **Most pizzas**

Pizza is one of the most popular snacks in the world. Most commercial pizzas are made with unhealthy ingredients, including the highly refined dough and highly processed meat. Pizza is relatively high in calories.

Alternatives

Some restaurants offer healthier ingredients. Homemade pizzas can also be very healthy, as long as you choose healthy ingredients.

3. **White bread**

Most commercial bread are unhealthy when eaten in large quantities because they are made from refined wheat, which is low in fiber and essential nutrients and can lead to rapid increases in blood sugar

Alternatives

For people who can tolerate gluten, Ezekiel bread is a great choice. Wholemeal bread is also healthier than white bread. If you have problems with gluten or carbohydrates, here are 15 bread recipes that are gluten-free and low in carbohydrates.

4.Most fruit juices

Fruit juice is often considered healthy. While the juice has some antioxidants and vitamin C, it also contains high amounts of liquid sugar. Fruit juice contains as much sugar as sugary drinks such as cola or digestion and sometimes even more (11).

Alternatives

Despite their sugar content, some fruit juices have health benefits, such as pomegranate juice and cranberry juice. However, these should be considered as supplements and not a daily part of your diet.

5.Sweet cereals

Breakfast cereals are processed grains such as wheat, oats, rice, and corn. They are especially popular with children and are often eaten with milk. To make them more delicious, the beans are baked, sliced, pulverized, wrapped, or peeled. They are generally high in sugar. The main disadvantage of most breakfast cereals is their high sugar content. Some are so sweet that they can even be compared to candy.

Alternatives

Choose breakfast cereals that are high in fiber and low in sugar. Make your oatmeal from scratch.

6. **Fried, grilled**

Baking, grilling, and baking are some of the most unhealthy cooking methods.

Food cooked this way is often very tasty and low in calories. Different types of unhealthy chemicals are also formed when food is cooked at a high temperature.

These include acrylamides, acrolein, heterocyclic amines, oxysterols, polycyclic aromatic hydrocarbons (PAHs) and advanced glycosylation end products (AGEs)

Many chemicals formed during high heat cooking have been linked to an increased risk of cancer and heart disease

Alternatives

Choose milder and healthier cooking methods, such as cooking, stew, bleaching, and steaming, to improve your health.

7. **Pastries, cookies, and cakes**

Most pastries, cookies, and cakes are unhealthy if eaten too much. Some packets are generally produced with refined sugar, wheat, flour, and additional fats. Shortness of breath is sometimes added, which can contain a lot of unhealthy trans fats. These delicacies can be delicious, but they contain almost no essential nutrients, many calories, and many preservatives.

Alternatives

If you can not stay away from dessert, go for Greek yogurt, fresh fruit, or dark chocolate.

8. French fries and potatoes

While white potatoes are very healthy. However, the same cannot be said for bands and brands. These foods are high in calories and easy to eat in excess. Several studies have linked potatoes and chips to weight gain These foods may also contain high amounts of acrylamides, which are carcinogenic that form, when potatoes are fried, fried or baked

Alternatives

Potatoes are best eaten cooked, not fried. If you need something crunchy to replace the chips, try carrots or walnuts.

9. Gluten-free snack

Some persons often replace healthy gluten with foods and processed junk foods that appear to be gluten-free. These gluten-free substitutes often contain a lot of sugar and refined grains such as cornstarch or tapioca starch. These ingredients can cause rapid increases in blood sugar and are low in essential nutrients.

Alternatives

Select foods that are normally gluten-free, such as unrefined Herbal and animal meals.

10. Agave nectar

A sweetener like an Agave nectar is often sold as healthy. However, it is very refined and extremely rich in fructose. High levels of fructose from added sweeteners can be completely detrimental to health In fact, agave nectar is even higher in fructose than many other sweeteners. While table sugar is 50% fructose and high fructose corn syrup is about 55%, agave nectar is 85% fructose (27).

Alternatives

Stevia and erythritol are natural, calorie-free, and healthy.

11. Low-fat yogurt

Yogurt can be incredibly healthy. However, most supermarket yogurts are bad for you. They are often low in fat but are contain much sugar to garnish the taste of fat. Simply put, most yogurts have replaced healthy, natural fats with an unhealthy ingredient. Besides, many yogurts do not contain probiotic bacteria as is generally believed. They are often pasteurized, killing most of their bacteria.

Alternatives

Choose plain, high-fat yogurt with live or active crops (probiotics). If possible, buy grass-fed cow breeds.

12. **Low carb junk food**

Low carb diets are very popular. While you can eat a lot of whole foods with such a diet, watch out for processed low carb substitutes. These include low carb candies and meal replacements. These foods are often highly processed and packaged with additives.

Alternatives

If you are on a low carb diet, aim for foods that are naturally low in carbohydrates, such as eggs, seafood, and leafy vegetables.

13. **Ice**

Ice cream can be delicious, but it is full of sugar. This dairy food is high in calories sometimes overeat. When you eat it for dessert, you usually put it above the normal calorie intake. Alternatives, you can choose healthier brands or make your ice cream with fresh fruit and less sugar.

14. Candies

The candies are incredibly unhealthy. They are high in sugar, refined wheat flour, and processed fats, and are also low in essential nutrients. Also, these treats will leave you hungry for the way your body metabolizes these sugar bombs. Instead, eat fruit or a high-quality piece of dark chocolate.

15. Processed meat

Although raw meat can be healthy and nutritious, this does not apply to cold cuts. Studies show that people who eat processed meats are at greater risk for many serious conditions, such as colon cancer, type 2 diabetes and heart disease Most of these studies are observational, which means that they cannot prove that processed meat is wrong. However, the statistical relationship is strong and consistent between the studies. Alternatives, if you want to eat bacon, sausages, or pepperoni, try buying from local butchers who do not add many unhealthy ingredients.

16. Processed cheese

The cheese is healthy in moderation. It is full of nutrients and a single slice packs all the nutrients like a glass of milk. However, processed cheese products do not look like ordinary cheese. They are usually made with filters designed to have a cheese-like appearance and texture. Be sure to read the labels to confirm that your cheese contains dairy products and some artificial ingredients.

Alternatively, eat real cheese. Healthy varieties include feta, mozzarella, and cottage cheese. Many alternatives to vegan cheese can also be good choices.

17. Most fast-food meals

Fast-food chains generally serve junk food. Most of their supply is mass-produced and low in nutrients. Despite their low prices, fast food can contribute to the risk of disease and harm your overall well-being. You should pay special attention to fried items.

Alternatively, as a result of increasing pressure, many fast-food chains have begun to offer healthy options.

18. High-calorie coffee drinks

Coffee is full of antioxidants and has many benefits. Coffee drinkers, in particular, have a lower risk of serious diseases such as type 2 diabetes and Parkinson's disease At the same time, creams, syrups, additives and sugars that are often added to coffee are very unhealthy. These products are just as harmful as any other sugary drink.

Alternatives

Drink regular coffee. If you want, you can add small amounts of whipped cream or whole milk. Anything with added sugar or refined grains It is important to avoid or at least limit foods that contain added sugar, refined grains, and artificial trans fats. These are some of the most unhealthy but common ingredients in the modern diet. Therefore, the importance of reading labels cannot be overstated.

Alternatives

Aim for nutritious, whole foods, such as fresh fruit and whole grains.

20. Most processed foods

The easiest way to eat and lose weight healthily is to avoid processed foods as much as possible. Processed products are often packaged and loaded with excess salt or sugar.

Alternatives

Make sure you read the food labels when shopping. Try to load your shopping cart with lots of vegetables and other whole foods.

NEVERTHELESS

While the western diet is high in junk food, if you keep the processed, sugary foods listed above, you can eat a healthy diet. If you focus on whole foods, you are ready to feel better and regain your health. Besides, exercising attention while eating by listening to your body signals and paying attention to flavors and textures can help you become more aware of how much and what you are eating, helping you to have a better relationship with food.

CHAPTER TEN

FOOD TO CONSUME MOST

HEALTHFUL FOODS YOU HAVE TO KNOW

It is important to know the healthiest foods to ensure a wide variety of nutrients in the diet. A balanced diet is a secret to a healthy diet. This book covers the 15 healthiest foods and their benefits.

Nuts, legumes, and cereals are very nutritious. The following are some of the healthiest

Almonds

Almonds are high in many nutrients, such as:

Magnesium, Vitamin E., iron, calcium, fiber, and riboflavin. Recent research found that consuming almonds significantly reduced total cholesterol levels.

Brazilian peanuts

Brazil nuts are some of the healthiest available nuts. They are a good product of protein and carbohydrates. They contain good amounts of vitamin E, magnesium, zinc, and vitamin B-1,. Brazil seeds also contain enough selenium than some other foods. Selenium is an essential metal for maintaining thyroid function and is an excellent antioxidant for the human body. These nuts come in a hard shell and are usually available ready-made, making them a quick, nutritious snack.

Lentils

Lentils are a pulse that is evident in many food crops around the world, including those of Pakistan, Nepal, Bangladesh, India, Bhutan, and Sri Lanka. Lentils provide good amounts of fiber, magnesium, and potassium. They usually require a long cooking time. However, manufacturers can germinate the seeds, making them a tasty, healthy, ready-to-eat snack. Adding a cup of sprouted lentils to a food box or picnic basket, perhaps with some chili powder or pepper to taste, creates a delicious and healthy snack.

HEALTH BENEFIT OF LENTILS

Lentils are an abundant source of fiber, folic acid, and potassium. These nutrients support heart health. According to recent research increased fiber intake can lower-density lipoprotein (LDL) cholesterol (LDL) cholesterol levels. Not only is fiber associated with a lower incidence of cardiovascular disease, but it can also slow the progression of the disease in high-risk individuals. Lentils add vital minerals, fiber, and vitamins, to the food. They also provide protein and are an excellent substitute for meat in meals. When a person replaces meat in the diet with foods rich in fiber, such as lentils, they reduce the risk of heart disease. Studies have shown that potassium, calcium, and magnesium in lentils can naturally lower blood pressure. Foods rich in these minerals are an important part of the DASH diet program. This diet lower blood pressure.

Oatmeal

Due to its health benefits, interest in oatmeal has grown significantly over the past 20 years.

Research has shown that the soluble fiber content of the grain helps lower cholesterol and cardiovascular risk factors. Oats contain complex carbohydrates and water-soluble fiber. These slow down digestion and help stabilize blood sugar. Oats are also a good source of folic acid and potassium. People can make oatmeal from oats. Coarse or steel oats contain more fiber than the immediate varieties.

Wheat germ

Wheat germ is an aspect that grows into a plant. It is essentially the embryo of a seed. Sprout, along with bran, is a by-product of the mill. Grain refining often removes germ and bran. However, whole grain products still contain germ and bran. This makes them a healthier choice. Wheat germ contains many essential nutrients, such as fiber, Vitamin E, folic acid, thiamine, zinc, magnesium, phosphorus, fatty alcohols, and essential fatty acids

Fruits, vegetables, and berries

Fruits, vegetables, and berries are easy to include in the diet. Here are some of the healthiest:

Broccoli

Broccoli provides good amounts of fiber, calcium, potassium, folic acid, and phytonutrients. Phytonutrients are compounds that reduce the risk of heart disease, diabetes, and certain cancers. Broccoli also contains essential antioxidants such as vitamin C and beta carotene. A serving of half a cup of broccoli can provide about 85% of a person's daily value of vitamin C.

Another substance in broccoli, called sulfonic Phane, may have anti-cancer and anti-inflammatory properties, according to a 2019 study. However, cooked broccoli can destroy many of its main nutrients. For this reason, it is best to eat it raw or lightly steamed.

Health Benefit Of Broccoli

Broccoli is rich in antioxidants, minerals, and vitamins. Antioxidants can help prevent the development of various conditions. The body produces molecules called free radicals during natural processes such as metabolism, and environmental stress adds up. Free radicals or reactive oxygen species are toxic in large quantities. They can cause cell damage that can lead to cancer and other conditions. The body can erase many of them, nevertheless, dietary antioxidants can assist.

Reduce the risk of cancer

Cross vegetables contain several antioxidants, which can help prevent the type of cell damage that leads to cancer. One is sulfonic Phane, a sulfur-containing compound that gives cruciferous vegetables their bitter bite. Some scientists have suggested that cruciferous vegetables such as broccoli may play a role in "green chemoprophylaxis", where people use the whole plant or extracts from it to help prevent cancer.

Cruciferous vegetables also contain indole-3-carbinol. 2019 research shows that this compound may have strong anti-cancer properties. Cauliflower, Brussels sprouts, cabbage, turnips, cabbage, arugula, broccoli, daikon, turnip, and cardamom all have similar properties.

Improving bone health

Calcium and collagen work together to build strong bones. More than 99% of the calcium in the body is in the bones and teeth. Also, the body needs vitamin C to generate collagen. Both are present in broccoli. Vitamin K plays a role in blood clotting, but some experts have also suggested that it may help prevent or treat osteoporosis. People with low vitamin K levels are more likely to have bone formation problems. Getting enough vitamin K from your diet can help keep your bones healthy.

According to recent research, a cup of broccoli weighing about 76 grams (g) contains 3% to 3.5% of a person's daily requirement of calcium, 45-54% of the daily requirement of vitamin C and 64 -86% of their daily needs for vitamin K, depending on their age and gender.

Improve the health of the immune system

Vitamin C is an antioxidant that offers many benefits. It supports the immune system and can help prevent cancer, cardiovascular disease (CVD), cataracts, and anemia. As a supplement, it can also help reduce the symptoms of the common cold and reduce the duration of the common cold.

Improve skin health

Vitamin C helps the body produce collagen, the body's main support system for cells and organs, including the skin. As an antioxidant, vitamin C can also help prevent skin damage, including wrinkles from aging. Studies have shown that vitamin C may play a role in preventing or treating skin conditions such as shingles and skin cancer.

Promoting digestion

Fiber can promote normalcy, prevent constipation, maintain a healthy digestive tract, and reduce the risk of colon cancer. In 2015, a screening study found that people who consumed the highest amount of fiber were less likely to develop colon cancer than those who consumed less fiber. A 76 g cup of broccoli provides 5.4% to 7.1% of a person's daily fiber requirement.

Reduce inflammation

When the immune system is affected, inflammation can occur. Inflammation can be a sign of a transient infection, but it can also occur in chronic autoimmune diseases such as arthritis and type 1 diabetes. People with metabolic syndrome may also have high levels of inflammation.

Broccoli can have anti-inflammatory effects, according to a 2014 study. Scientists have found that the antioxidant activity of sulforaphane in broccoli helped reduce inflammation markers in laboratory tests. They, therefore, concluded that the nutrients in broccoli can help fight inflammation.

Reduce the risk of diabetes

A 2017 study showed that eating broccoli can help people with type 2 diabetes control their blood sugar. This is due to the sulforaphane content.

Protection of cardiovascular health

A 2018 population study found that older women whose diet was high in cruciferous vegetables had a lower risk of atherosclerosis. This is a condition of the blood vessels that can lead to a heart attack or stroke. This benefit may be due to the antioxidant content of cruciferous vegetables, especially sulforaphane.

One cup of broccoli provides almost 5% of your daily potassium needs.

Apples

Apples are an excellent source of antioxidants that fight free radicals. Free radicals are harmful substances produced by the body. They cause unwanted changes in the body and can contribute to chronic diseases and the aging process. However, some studies have shown that an antioxidant in apples can extend a person's lifespan and reduce the risk of chronic disease.

Health Benefit

Apples are rich in fiber, vitamins, and minerals, which all benefit health. They also offer a variety of antioxidants. These substances help to neutralize free radicals.

Free radicals are reactive molecules that can accumulate as a result of natural processes and environmental stress. If too many free radicals accumulate in the body, they can cause oxidative stress, which can lead to cell damage. This damage can contribute to several conditions, including cancer and diabetes. Apples contain several antioxidants, such as quercetin, catechin, fluoride, chlorogenic acid, etc

Neurological health and dementia

A 2019 laboratory study concluded that quercetin has a neuroprotective effect, possibly because it prevents the formation of reactive species. It seems to help neurons survive and continue to function. It can, therefore, help prevent age-related neuronal loss. In 2015, the results of a mouse study showed that supplementation with a high dose of quercetin can help protect cells from the type of damage that can lead to Alzheimer's disease. It is worth noting that most studies of this type have used high doses of quercetin that are unlikely to be present in normal dietary sources. Besides, scientists need to do more human studies to confirm that quercetin improves neurological health in humans.

Stroke

An earlier study from 2000 looked at how eating apples for 28 years affected the risk of stroke in 9,208 people. The authors found that those who ate the most apples had a lower risk of thrombosis. Apples are high in nutrients that can reduce the risk of stroke. For example, a 2017 review found that people who consume the most fiber seem to have a lower risk of cardiovascular disease, coronary heart disease, and stroke.

Kale

Kale is a green, leafy vegetable that offers a wide variety of different nutrients. For example, this powerful nutrient plant is an excellent source of vitamins C and K. People can cook or curl up. They can also be mixed into smoothies or juices for a nutritious kick.

A medium-sized apple about 3 inches in diameter and weighing 182 grams (g) provides 4.37 g of fiber. This is about 13-20% of an adult's daily needs, depending on their age and gender.

Health Benefit

Kale contains fiber, antioxidants, calcium, vitamins C and K, iron, and a wide variety of other nutrients that can help prevent various health problems. Antioxidants help the body get rid of unwanted toxins that result from natural processes and environmental pressure. These toxins, also known as free radicals, are unstable molecules. If too much is built up in the body, they can lead to cell damage. This can lead to health problems such as inflammation and disease. Experts believe that, for example, free radicals can play a role in the development of cancer.

Diabetes

The American Diabetes Association recommends consuming foods rich in vitamins, minerals, fiber, and antioxidants. There is some evidence that some of these offer protection against diabetes. Fiber: A 2018 study concluded that people who consume the highest amounts of dietary fiber appear to have a lower risk of developing type 2 diabetes. Consuming dietary fiber can also lower blood sugar, the authors note.

Several nutrients in kale can support heart health.

Potassium: Potassium intake will reduce the consumption of added salt or sodium. It also can reduce the risk of high blood pressure and cardiovascular disease. A cup of cooked kale provides 3.6% of an adult's daily potassium requirement.

Fiber: A 2016 Cochrane review found a link between fiber consumption and lower blood fat and blood pressure. People who consumed more fiber were more likely to have lower total cholesterol and low-density lipoprotein (LDL) or `` bad " cholesterol. Humans need both soluble and insoluble fiber.

Cancer: Kale and many green vegetables contain chlorophyll which can assist prevent the body from absorbing heterocyclic amines. These chemicals occur when people grill the food of animals at a high temperature. Experts have linked them to cancer. The human body cannot absorb much chlorophyll, but chlorophyll binds to these carcinogens and prevents the body from absorbing them. In this way, kale can reduce cancer risk, and combining a grilled steak with green vegetables can help reduce the negative impact.

Antioxidants: Vitamin C, beta carotene, selenium, and other antioxidants in kale can help prevent cancer. Studies have not shown that supplements have the same effect, but people with a high intake of fruits and vegetables seem to have a lower risk of developing various cancers. This may be due to the antioxidants these foods contain.

Bone health: healthy bone formation is strong with the assistance of Calcium and phosphorus. Some studies have suggested that high vitamin K intake may help reduce the risk of bone fractures. A cup of cooked kale provides nearly five times an adult's daily requirement of vitamin K, about 15-18% of his calcium requirement, and about 7% of daily phosphorus requirement.

Digestion: Kale is high in water and fiber, which supports the prevention of constipation and promote regularity and a healthy digestive tract.

Skin and hair: Kale is a good source of beta carotene, the carotenoid that the body converts to vitamin A as needed. Beta carotene and vitamin A are necessary for the growth and maintenance of all body tissues, including the skin and hair. The body uses vitamin C to make and maintain collagen, a protein that provides the structure for skin, hair, and bones. Vitamin C is also in kale. A cup of cooked kale provides at least 20% of a person's daily requirement of Vitamin A and more 23% of all supplements contain vitamin C.

Eye health: Kale contains lutein and zeaxanthin, a combination of antioxidants that can help reduce the risk of age-related macular degeneration. Vitamin C, vitamin E, β-carotene, and zinc also play a role in eye health.

Blackberries

Cranberries contain significant amounts of fiber, antioxidants, and phytonutrients. Unlike minerals and vitamins, phytonutrients are not essential for survival. However, they can help prevent disease and maintain vital bodily functions.

Quick facts about cranberries

Cranberries can be eaten fresh or incorporated into a variety of recipes. They can also be purchased frozen. Cranberries contain a plant compound called anthocyanin. This gives blackberries both their blue color and many of their health benefits. Cranberries can help with heart, bone, skin health, blood pressure, diabetes management, cancer prevention, and mental health. One cup of blueberries provides 24% of the recommended daily allowance of vitamin C.

Use blueberries to cover waffles, pancakes, yogurt, oatmeal, or cereal, mix them into a smoothie or syrup or fold them into muffins and sweet buns. People taking blood thinners, such as warfarin, should talk to their doctor before increasing their blueberry intake, as high vitamin K levels can affect blood clotting.

Health Benefit

Maintaining healthy bones: Blueberries contain iron, phosphorus, calcium, magnesium, manganese, zinc, and vitamin K. Each of them is part of the bones. Adequate intake of these minerals and vitamins helps build and maintain bone structure and strength. Iron and zinc play a key role in maintaining the strength and elasticity of bones and joints. Low vitamin K intake has been linked to a higher risk of bone fractures. However, adequate vitamin K intake improves calcium absorption and can reduce calcium loss.

Skin health: Collagen is the skin support system. It is based on vitamin C as a key nutrient and helps prevent skin damage from the sun, pollution, and smoke. Vitamin C can also improve the ability of collagen to smooth out wrinkles and improve the overall texture of the skin. One cup of blueberries provides 24% of the recommended daily allowance of vitamin C.

Reduction of blood pressure

Maintaining a low sodium level is essential to keeping blood pressure at a healthy level. Cranberries do not contain sodium. They contain potassium, calcium, and magnesium. Some studies have found that diets low in minerals are associated with higher blood pressure. Adequate nutritional intake of these minerals would help lower blood pressure.

However, other studies refute these findings. For example, a 2015 study in people with metabolic syndrome found that daily consumption of raspberries for 6 weeks did not affect blood pressure.

Diabetes management

Studies have shown that people with type 1 diabetes who eat high-fiber diets have low blood sugar levels and those with type 2 diabetes who eat the same may have improved blood sugar, lipid, and insulin levels. One cup of blueberries provides 3.6 grams (g) of fiber.

Researchers found that consuming three servings a week of blueberries, grapes, raisins, apples, or pears reduced the risk of type 2 diabetes by 7%.

Protection against heart disease

Blueberries can help maintain cardiovascular health. The content of fiber, potassium, folic acid, vitamin C, vitamin B6, and phytonutrients in blueberries supports heart health. Lack of raspberry cholesterol is also beneficial for the heart. Fiber helps reduce the amount of cholesterol in the blood and reduces the risk of heart disease.

Vitamin B6 and folic acid prevent the accumulation of a compound known as homocysteine. Excessive accumulation of homocysteine in the body can damage blood vessels and lead to heart problems.

Frequent intake of anthocyanins can decrease the risk of heart attack by 32% in infants and middle-aged women. The study found that women who ate at least three servings of raspberries or strawberries a week showed the best results.

Cancer prevention

Vitamin C, vitamin A and various phytonutrients in blackberries act as powerful antioxidants that can help protect cells from disease-related free radical damage. Research shows that antioxidants can inhibit tumor growth, reduce inflammation in the body, and prevent or delay cancer of the esophagus, lung, mouth, throat, endometrium, pancreas, prostate, and colon. Cranberries also contain folic acid, which plays a role in DNA synthesis and repair. This can prevent the formation of cancer cells due to mutations in DNA.

Improving mental health

Population studies have shown that raspberry consumption is associated with slower cognitive decline in older women. Studies have also shown that blueberries not only reduce the risk of cognitive impairment but can also improve a person's short-term memory and motor coordination.

Healthy digestion, weight loss and feeling full

Cranberries help prevent constipation and maintain a normal digestive tract due to its fiber content. Dietary fiber is also widely recognized as an important factor in weight loss weight management by acting as a "filler" in the digestive system. Foods high in fiber increase satiety or a feeling of fullness and reduce appetite.

Avocado

Some people avoid avocados because of their high-fat content. However, avocados provide healthy fats, as do B vitamins, vitamin K and vitamin E. Avocados are also a good source of fiber. In a review of 2018 studies, avocados increased levels of high-density lipoprotein or good cholesterol. This type of cholesterol removes more harmful cholesterol from the bloodstream. Avocados can also have anti-cancer properties. A study of avocado test tubes from 2019 showed that colored avocado seed extract reduced the viability of breast, colon, and prostate cancer cells. However, the study did not show whether the effects would be the same in humans. Avocados may also be associated with improved nutrient absorption, better overall nutrition, and fewer metabolic risk factors, according to a 2013 study. Avocados are very nutritious and very full.

Pineapple

My first choice is Pineapple. Pineapple bioflavonoid bromelain is a proteolytic enzyme (meaning it breaks down proteins). It is believed to enhance immune function and has anti-inflammatory properties that help open the airways. In nutritional medicine, bromelain is often used to support sinus disease (reduces swelling and mucus production) and helps clear both the upper and lower respiratory tract.

Other fruits that I like to support the immune system are berries and citrus fruits, especially grapefruit. Grapefruit is ideal for breaking down excess mucus and is now happy in season. I also like lemon or lime juice in hot water for hydration which helps eliminate mucus and supports immune function. This immune tea recipe is also a favorite.

Green leafy vegetables

A 2019 study in rats found that eating leafy green vegetables for 6 weeks significantly reduced cardiovascular risk factors.

Spinach is an example of leafy greens with antioxidant content, especially when cooked raw, steamed, or lightly cooked. It is a good source of the following nutrients: Vitamins A, B-6, C, E and K., selenium, nicotinic acid, zinc,

Phosphorus, Copper, Potassium, Calcium, Manganese, Betaine, and iron.

Sweet potatoes

Sweet potatoes contain fiber, vitamin A, vitamin C, vitamin B-6, and potassium.

The Science Center for the Public Interest compared the nutritional value of sweet potatoes with that of many other vegetables. Sweet potatoes came first because of their content of vitamin A, vitamin C, iron, calcium, protein, and complex carbohydrates.

Fish, meat and eggs

When it comes to fish, meat, and eggs, there are many healthy options.:

Fatty fish

Some examples of fatty fish are salmon, trout, mackerel, herring, sardines, and anchovies. These species of fish have oil in their tissues and around their intestines. Their lean fillets are high in omega-3 fatty acids. These oils can provide benefits to the heart and nervous system, according to research. Omega-3 fatty acids may help with inflammatory conditions such as arthritis. They are also rich in vitamins A and D.

Chicken

Chicken is cost-effective and healthy meat. Chicken is a good means of protein. However, it is important to remember that cooking methods affect how healthy the chicken is. This means that people should limit their intake of fried chicken and always remove the skin before eating. Because a lot of fat is in the Chicken skin.

Eggs

Eggs are another source of protein that people can easily incorporate into a balanced diet because they are so versatile.

Eggs contain vitamins, including B-2 and B-12, both of which are important for maintaining energy and building red blood cells. Eggs are also a good source of the essential amino acid leucine, which plays a role in stimulating the synthesis of muscle proteins. Eggs also provide a good amount of choline, which is important for cell membranes. The yolk contains most of the vitamins and minerals in the egg, as well as fat and cholesterol. However, a 2017 review found that eating up to seven eggs a week does not increase the risk of heart disease. However, People with cardiovascular disease or diabetes should seek medical advice about including eggs in their diet. Indeed, one study found a higher rate of cardiovascular disease in people who consumed more cholesterol than eggs. Consuming fat in moderation is healthy as part of a balanced, nutritious diet.

CHAPTER ELEVEN

DISCIPLINE FOR GOOD HEALTH

IMPORTANCE OF GOOD HEALTH

1. Helps you stop eating unhealthy foods

Eating too much, eating junk food, and eating too much sugar is not good for your health. A large number of people have no control over their food due to a lack of discipline. They just can't change their eating habits because they don't have the inner strength to do so.

If they had some discipline, they could have reduced the amount of food they ate, avoided junk food, and consumed less sugar. This would improve their health and prevent any kind of health problem.

2. Helps you reduce the amount of alcohol you drink. Drinking a cup or two of alcohol can be okay for most people. However, when drinking becomes a habit over which you have no control, it becomes a problem. Having self-discipline can help you to resist alcohol consumption without restrictions. Of course, you need to develop this ability before you become a heavy drinker. Then it would be easier to resist the temptation to drink too much. A heavy drinker can find it difficult to show discipline and therefore needs extra resources and help. However, a large number of people who do not drink a lot of alcohol would find that having a certain degree of discipline is very helpful in controlling this habit.

3. Helps you avoid drugs

People who use drugs know that it is not good for their health and that they can harm it, but due to lack of discipline, they can not stop using it. If there was a way to improve their discipline, they could be done to reduce their use and even stop using it. A person who does not use drugs and works to educate and improve self-discipline is more likely to abstain and abstain from drugs.

4. Allows you to exercise your body

Do you avoid physical activity? Would you rather lie down on your couch, watch TV and eat a snack when you get home from work?

You keep telling yourself you're going to the gym next week, but does that never happen?

If you develop even a little self-discipline, you can let yourself go to the gym, walk or exercise your body regularly with any kind of sport. Doing exercise regularly is essential for your health. If you have discipline, you will not succumb to laziness and procrastination. It gives you the strength and determination to decide to exercise your body and make that decision.

5. **Helps you lose weight**

How many persons are you aware of who tried to scale down weight but could not follow their decisions? You may have tried to lose weight, but you could not resist the delicious food, the tempting cakes, or the delicious ice cream. You may have tried different diets, but stopped after a week or two. What stopped you from losing weight? There is a lack of discipline and self-control. Imagine how much leaner you can be if you are in control of the amount of food you eat and you could follow your diet until you lose weight. Some industries can help you lose weight.

6. Helps you quit smoking

Smoking is an unhealthy habit, most smokers have often thought about quitting, but could not. They may say that they control this habit and can stop it whenever they want, but they do not do it because they do not have enough will and inner strength. If you want to improve your discipline, it is easier to quit smoking.

7. Allows you to control your anger

Anger is not good for your health. It has negative effects on the mind and body, increases blood pressure, and causes stress. You should avoid getting angry, arguing, or raising your voice or showing verbal or physical aggression. To do this you need discipline and inner strength.

8. Makes it possible to avoid impulsive and thoughtless

Impulsivity means a lack of control and action without thought. If you do not have control over your actions and the words you say, you may run into problems and sometimes dangerous situations. A little discipline will reduce impulsivity, add common sense, and help you avoid stress and unnecessary risks.

Printed in Great Britain
by Amazon